Bitter Sweet Herbals

Home Remedies
and
First Aid Medicine

Davilyn Atwood

Table of Contents

Introduction

Welcome to the world of learning how to create and use herbals in your own home. I hope that you will find this book a daily help. You will find information all about herbs, their properties, their nutritional value, and how to use them. There are also many great recipes for healing, body care, and eating!

My home apothecary is growing and expanding on a daily basis. The generations to follow are showing great interest also as they see the amazing benefits that come from using nature at it's finest.

In the second part of Bitter Sweet Herbals, you will find great information to help you with your herbal first aid needs, with great advice and many remedies and recipes!

Blessings to you on your journey!

Apothecary

Apothecary- that is what they used to call someone who would create remedies and dispense medicines to those who needed them. Apotheca, means a place where wine, spices and herbs were stored. Apothecary came to mean the person who would stock these and often offer general medical advice, and sometimes even offered some basic medical services.

"The word apothecary, in the Norman period of English history, designated anyone who kept a shop or store of such nonperishable commodities as spices, drugs, comfits and preserves. During the later Middle Ages, the term was restricted to those who prepared and sold drugs. Not until the end of the 18th century were the professions of apothecary and physician clearly distinguished." Harold B. Gill, Jr., The Apothecary in Colonial Virginia.

Everywhere in the world throughout time, herbs have been an integral part of human life. People grew and gathered herbs because of their powerful medicinal and nutritive properties. India has used ginger, pepper, and mustard in Ayurveda medicine for 6,000 years. Chinese medicine has used herbs like ginseng and angelica for 3,000 years or longer. Hippocrates said, "Healing is a matter of time, but it is also sometimes also a matter of opportunity." Herbs offer that opportunity in all cultures throughout all of history, including our modern medicine.

I personally love the pictures of the old time apothecaries that we see. I can imagine as I walk into that old time shop, the smell of something brewing, and all of the antique jars, containers and labels. The blends of spices and colourful containers full of all types of herbs and spices. It is a dimly lit place with an old wooden floor. There is an older gentleman behind the counter grinding up some herbs with his mortar and pestle, with his apprentice faithfully standing by to learn every little detail. It is quite the lovely picture in my mind - simple, pure, and of the earth. Oh the simple life!

These apothecary shops would often consist of three rooms. One would be the main store with shelves full of antique jars, prepared remedies, herbs, and spices. The second room might be like the lab or kitchen, where the preparation of the remedies would take place. And if there were a third room, it likely would have been a room used for consulting with customers or patients. The apothecary garden plot was located in the back yard, where the herbs would be growing that were used in the remedies. This apothecary could identify all of the plants, and describe how to use each of them. He knew the details of many, many different materials and it was his job to make sure you got the right thing for the right symptom.

One of America's oldest botanical garden was created in 1728 by John Bartram. It includes many varieties from old apothecary gardens, as well as new world herbs. This garden is a living museum today, and features various theme gardens like: kitchen gardens, herb gardens, and medicinal gardens. "whatsoever whether great or small, ugly or handsome sweet or stinking…everything in the universe in their own nature appears beautiful to me." John Bartram, 1740. John Bartram was America's first botanist, and was curious in wanting to learn everything about the world around him.

A Gingko Biloba tree, in Vancouver, B.C. is believed to be the oldest one in North America. It was one of the original trees brought from London in 1785. Vancouver, British Columbia in Canada, hosts the oldest botanical garden in Canada. It contains five gardens and is spread over 70 acres of land. One of its gardens is the Physick Garden, which is recreated to represent a 16th century monastery herb garden. It is grown in raised brick beds, with traditional plants that are all used for medicinal purposes.

The Chelsea Physic Garden. It is the oldest surviving garden of it's type. These types of gardens were called physic gardens and were training ground for apothecary apprentices. These weren't created to be pretty gardens, but were practical and functional. The apothecary and his apprentice would have such a garden as this and each section of the garden would contain herbs for specific symptoms or aliments. The Chelsea Physic Garden
Diseases used to be classified as symptoms. The apothecary would work with the symptoms

of the patients and would prescribe a remedy that would work for a specific symptom. An apprentice would usually get into this profession by showing interest in what the apothecary was doing, or by having an interest in plants and herbs. Often today, this is still how herbalists and other natural types of medical professions learn, by someone who has already learned the ways, and is training apprentices. And of course by reading lots of books. It is always a good idea to have a library of reliable books on hand that you know in and out and can reference quickly.

Apothecaries have evolved into what we have today as pharmacies. In the early 19th century scientist began to study the properties of plants. They began to understand the active ingredients of the plants and how they work with the body. Thus developed the modern day pharmacies that we have today. Over 80 percent of the world today still used herbal remedies, but in our modernized society, we have come to rely on the pharmaceutical companies to prescribe chemical remedies. Unfortunately these drugs often have horrible side effects that can sometimes be worse than the original symptoms. This has created a movement within our culture to get back to natural health. We see health food stores everywhere now, and more and more people are studying alternate medicines with hopes to get back to healing our bodies without the use of drugs. Pills, tinctures, lotions, essential oils, teas, and so many other kinds of remedies are readily available. These more closely resemble the apothecary of old, minus the apprentice and the teacher.

There are those of us who want to keep this art of old world medicine alive, and have decided to pass it along to the next generation. And in this process of my attempting to keep it alive, I have come across some things that are just essential in my home apothecary. There are some herbs that are must haves, and some that are good to haves. There are some essential oils that are must haves also. There are also many other basic products that are essential to make the remedies. An apothecary doesn't just consist of herbal products, there are also tools that are essential to make things work. In the following pages, we will cover the essentials of what your home apothecary should consist of, and some home remedies that are good to know and easy to make.

Having a knowledge of these things and a great collection of recipes and things that go into them, will allow you to create pretty much everything you need for the remedies you want. It will save you a lot of money in the long run after a few small investments. And to top it all off, it is fun and satisfying to know that you can create a remedy to solve a problem and heal someone.

I would suggest that you take it one step at a time as well. Don't just dive in and expect to do it all at once. Experiment with one or two herbs at a time. Test it in everything and every way. Learn all you can learn about that herb. The best way to do it is a little at a time, so you don't get overwhelmed.

The Herbs

Herbs come in all shapes, sizes, colors, scents, and properties. Sometimes it can be a bit overwhelming where to start. How do I know which herbs are the basics? Where do I even begin to learn? Well it really is a matter of personal preference. There are herbs that are going to grow locally, learn which ones they are, and what they can do for you. Don't try to learn everything about every herb. If you can master the knowledge of a few plants, you will learn that they can be used for multiple things.

Learn which part of the herbs to use, how to use it, and what it can be used for, and you are well on your way. Learning the locally grown herbs will save you money, as you can harvest for free.

If you are a beginner at herbs, it is probably best for you to do your practice with dried herbs. They are inexpensive and easy to come by. You will likely even start to grow some of your favorite herbs, but for now, dry herbs will serve the purpose for what you are learning. Growing herbs is actually pretty simple. And without a doubt, you will want to start growing them before too long. It will just be a logical next step.

It is important to purchase good quality organic herbs, from a reputable location. Your little health food store down the road may sell bulk herbs, but as I have found, they are not always the freshest, and they lose their potency after a time. I have found **Mountain Rose Herbs** to have great quality herbs, good prices, and they ship in a quick amount of time.
I am sure that there are many other great places to purchase dried herbs from, so do your homework and find a reputable source for your supplies.

One good thing to think about when storing your herbs is to not store them in clear jars, unless they are kept in a dark cupboard. The sunlight and other lighting will break down the properties of the herbs and they will be pretty much worthless and a waste of your purchase before too long. Keep them dry, and dark for the longest shelf life.

Herbal Properties

When you are starting out with herbs, it is important to understand their properties. I easily learned which herb to use for which ailment, but I didn't always understand the properties of the herbs and what each property meant. By knowing these properties of different herbs, it all makes so much more sense as to how many different ways you can be using a few simple herbs in your apothecary. The remarkable thing about herbs is that they contain several healing properties. The properties often combine to provide specific effects on certain systems of the body, which provides a quick overall healing. This can attack a disease and it symptoms, and your overall health, with minimal herbs being used, by understanding all of the properties of that certain herb.

Learn the properties of the herbs you love and you will be able to use them for many different things, according to how you prepare them.

The herbal property and what it does

- **Adaptogen** - nervine, helps support the nervous system, helps your body adapt to what it needs, aids in memory
- **Alteratives** - blood purifiers, help assimilate nutrition and eliminate waste
- **Analgesics** - pain relievers
- **Antacids** - neutralize acids in the stomach
- **Antiaboratives** - help inhibit abortive tendencies during
- **Antiasthmatics** - relieve the symptoms of asthma
- **Anti-emetic** - relieves vomiting, relieve nausea, travel and morning sickness
- **Antibiotics** - inhibits the growth of bacteria and viruses, enhances the immune system
- **Anticatarrhals** - dry up mucus
- **Anti-inflammatory** - reduce inflammation in the muscles
- **Antimicrobial** - directly kills pathogens or helps the immune system to kill them
- **Antipyretics** - cooling herbs for use with fevers
- **Anti puruitic** - reduces itching
- **Antiseptics** - applied to the skin to control bacteria growth
- **Antispasmodics** - helps relax muscles spasms
- **Anti-tussive** - cough suppressant
- **Aphrodisiacs** - enhances sexual potency and drive
- **Astringents** - have binding or constricting effect, tightens tissues, used to stop hemorrhaging or secretions, dries up wet conditions, can also dry up breast milk
- **Anxiolytic** - support coping for stress and anxiety, nervine tonics
- **Bitter** - promote production of bile, helps to increase appetite, tonics
- **Bronchial** - respiratory herbs, sooth lung tissues, ease coughs and congestion
- **Carminatives** - relieves gas, bloating, and indigestion
- **Cholagogues** - laxatives by promoting flow of bile
- **Demulcents** - smoothing, usually mucilage, protects damaged tissue
- **Diaphoretics** - induce sweating, some are relaxing and some are stimulating
- **Diuretics** - increase the flow of urine and reduce water retention
- **Emetics** - induce vomiting
- **Emmenagogues** - promote menstruation

- **Emollients** - soften and smooth the skin
- **Expectorants** - expel mucus from the lungs and throat
- **Febrifuge** - help break or reduce fevers, antipyretics
- **Galactagogues** - increase the production of milk for nursing mothers
- **Hemostatics** - stop hemorrhaging, styptics
- **Hepatic** - toning and supporting the liver
- **Inotropic** - increase contractility of the heart
- **Laxatives** - promote bowel movements
- **Lithotriptics** - help dissolve and remove kidney or other types of stones
- **Mucilaginous** - slimy, relieves hot and inflamed, cooling, soothing
- **Nervines** - calm nervousness and nourish the nervous system
- **Oxytocics** - stimulate uterine contractions and induce labor
- **Panacea** - heal all, cure all
- **Parasiticides** - destroy parasites in the digestive system
- **Purgatives** - laxatives, usually toxic, expel fluids from the body via urine, bowel, sweating
- **Rubefacients** - increase the flow of blood at the surface of the skin, drawing from deeper areas to promote healing
- **Sedatives** - induce relaxation and promote sleep
- **Sialogogues** - increase the flow of saliva and aid in digestion
- **Soporific** - strong sedatives
- **Stimulants** - increase the energies in the body and help to increase circulation
- **Stomachics** - help promote general body health, some are more system specific, taken long term
- **Styptics** - stop the blood flow to an area so it can scab, hemostatic
- **Tonics** - same as stomachics, nourishing, toning, calming, taken long term
- **Vermifuge** - expel worms
- **Vulneraries** - promotes healing of wounds, promotes cell growth and repair, mends broken things and skin

Herbs and Their Uses

Herbs, the parts used, their properties, and methods most often used

- **Ashwaghanda root** - tonic, sedative, antiflammatory, nervine, immune booster, aphrodisiac - general tonic or capsule

- **Astragalus root** - stimulant, immune booster, antioxidant, anti tumor, hepatic - capsule or tea

- **Balm of Gilead** resinous leaf bud - expectorant for upper respiratory, salve aches, salve for skin - cough syrup or salve

- **Bilberry** leaf and berry - astringent, hepatic, diuretic, good for eyes, helps reduce macular degeneration - pill form

- **Burdock** root, seeds, leaves - alterative, good for kidneys, diuretic, nutritive - teas and tonics

- **Calendula** flower heads - vulnerary, emollient, antibacterial, diaphoretic, alterative, astringent - oil or salve, poultice for skin, tea, great to use for varicose veins.

- **Cayenne** fruit - diaphoretic, expectorant, stimulant, rubefacient, anodyne, vasodilator, hypotensive, antimicrobial - food, capsule, salve

- **Chamomile** flower heads - nervine, tonic, sedative, antispasmodic, carminative, anti-inflammatory - tea, pill, salves

- **Charcoal** - activated - absorbent for toxins and poisons - pill, salves, or alone

- **Comfrey** leaf and root - tonic, fast healing, bone knit, demulcent, vulnerary, astringent, expectorant - tea, capsule, or salve, used to heal deep wounds / bones - not open wounds, assists with blood clotting,

- **Dandelion** whole plant - alterative, cholagogue, diuretic, stomachic, aperient, tonic, glactagogue, hepatic, tea for liver and organ problems and cleansing

- **Echinacea** root and leaves - antibacterial, febrifuge, immune stimulant, antiviral, anti-inflammatory, tonic, adaptogen, anticatarrhal - tea, tincture, capsule for respiratory infections and other infections also

- **Elderberries**, berry and flowers - stimulant, anticatarrhal, antirheumatic, alterative, diaphoretic, immune stimulant - teas or tinctures for colds, flu, fevers

- **Eyebright**, aerial portions - astringent, anti-inflammatory, expectorant - eyewash, tea for eyes and sinus
- **Feverfew**, whole herb - analgesic, anti-inflammatory, emmenagogue, purgative, carminative - capsule or tincture daily
- **Garlic** cloves - immune system builder, antioxidant, anti inflammatory, antifungal - capsule, tincture, cooking
- **Ginger**, rhizome - antiviral, sedative, analgesic - tea, capsule, tincture, or cooking
- **Gingko Biloba** leaves - vasoactive properties, cerebral, nervine, antioxidant, improves peripherial blood circulation, good for renyalds syndrome, adhd, alzheimers, etc - capsule
- **Ginseng Siberian** - Bark of root - **Eleuthero** - adaptogenic energy tonic, nervine, antirheumatic, antispasmodic, mild aphrodisiac - capsule, tincture, tea used for low energy as an energy boost
- **Hawthorn** berries, leaves, and flowers - cardiotonic, tonic, hypotensive, vasodilator, antioxidant - tea, capsule, or tincture
- **Kava Kava** root - antispasmodic, stimulant, intoxicant, diuretic, antifungal, muscle relaxant - tincture for mild tranquilizer, not long term use
- **Lavender** flowers - aromatic, nervine, sedative, carminative, antispasmodic, antidepressant, antispetic, vulnerary - tincture, salves, oil, lotion
- **Lemon Balm** leaves - nervine, vulnerary, antiviral, cerebral, vasodilator, hypotensive, antispasmodic, carminative - tea, tincture for fevers, depression, nerves, digestion
- **Marshmallow** root, leaf - emollient, demulcent, vulnerary, antibacterial - tea, poultice, capsule, tincture
- **Milk Thistle** leaf, flower - hepatic, bitter tonic, demulcent, antidepressant - tincture, protect and regenerate liver
- **Mullein** leaf, flower - expectorant, demulcent, antibacterial, antispasmodic, antitussive, astringent - tincture, smoke, tea, opens the bronchial tubes
- **Nettle** leaf, stem, root - tonic, diuretic, nutrient, histamine, rubefacient, hemostatic, laxative, hypotensive, galactagogue - nutritive, tea, capsule, tincture overall health, promotes healthy adrenal glands and kidneys, expels toxins, joint pain treatment
- **Passionflower** leaves - sedative, hypnotic, antispasmodic, anodyne, hypotensive - tincture, capsule, tea, for nerves or insomnia

- **Peppermint** leaves - carminative to nerves, stimulant to circulation, antispasmodic, stomachic, rubefacient - tea, essential oils
- **Plantain** leaves and seeds - diuretic, alterative, anti-inflammatory, aperient - tea for urinary, poultice for external wounds
- **Raspberry** leaf - hemostatic, astringent, mild alterative, parturient - tea for pregnancy and delivery, and menstrual problems
- **Skullcap** aerial portions - sedative, nervine, antispasmodic – tincture, tea, or capsule for nerves, insomnia, and with drawl symptoms from drugs or alcohol
- **St. John's Wort** herb - sedative, antidepressant, anti-inflammatory, astringent - tea, capsule, tincture for nerves, depression, insomnia
- **Stevia** leaves - sweetener, reduce blood glucose levels - use as a sweetener
- **Usnea** whole plant - antibiotic, antifungal, tuberculostatic – tincture, used as an atibiotic for fungal, viral, and bacterial infections
- **Uva Ursi** leaves - diuretic, urinary antiseptic, astringent - tea for urinary tract infections and problems
- **Valerian** rhizome - sedative, hypnotic, nervine, antispasmodic, carminative - tea, tincture or capsule for insomnia, stress, pain relief
- **Yarrow** herb - diaphoretic, anti-inflammatory, antipyreic, carminative, hemostatic, astringent - tea, tincture, or capsule for colds, fevers, bleeding and hemorrhoids

Whole Herb Tinctures

There are some good herbs to have on hand as individual tinctures. You can always combine them if you come across a recipe that calls for a blend.

Cayenne Pepper - good to help stop bleeding, fevers, varicose veins, asthma.

Dandelion root - brings quick relief to chronic inflammation of liver, relieves stomach cramps, helps to clear up skin rashes, among many other things. It is an all around nourishing tonic.

Nettle leaf - used for allergies, and anaemia. Great tonic and source of iron. Good for stimulating circulation.

Oregon Grape Root - great antiseptic and antibacterial, will lower fevers and fight infection, good liver tonic and detoxifier

Plantain herb - good for constipation or diarrhea. Use on bites and stings, including animal bites. Use on all external wounds. Good internal for asthma and bronchial

Skullcap herb - good tincture for nervous or anxiety, and insomnia. Best herb for with drawls from barbiturates and tranquilizers

St. John's wort - good for depression, anxiety, and nervous tension Good for shingles, bruises and injuries

Valerian - best for insomnia, anxiety, cramps, migraines, hypertension and painful menstruation

Wild yam root - used for irritable bowel syndrome, stomach complaints, morning sickness, painful menstruation, asthma and whooping cough

White Willow Bark - can replace aspirin for pain relief.

Yarrow flower and leaves - powerful healer and purifier, internally for fever and diarrhea and pretty much anything else. Yarrow is often considered a cure for all ills.

Herbal Nutrition

All too often the supplements that we purchase at the grocery store or pharmacy are full of synthetic ingredients, preservatives and neurotoxins. They don't contain a complete synergy that a whole plant offers.

Whole herbs offer a complete nutritious balance of vitamins and minerals in a form that is completely assimilable. No waste, no additives, no synthetics, no toxins. Herbs help our bodies to fight against toxins, germs and help to boost our immune system. They really are a medicine all to themselves.

Vitamins, Minerals and what they do:

Vitamin A - enhances immunity, support and prevents eye problems and skin disorders, slows ageing, good for bones and teeth

B1, Thiamine - improves mental attitude, strengthens nervous system, prevents stress

Riboflavin, B2 - red blood formation, hair, skin and nail growth, prevents cataracts

Niacin, B3 - proper circulation, increases energy, helps prevent migraines

B5, Panothenic Acid - enhance stamina, helps heal wounds, fight infection and strengthen immune

B6, Pyridoxine - absorption of fats and proteins, prevents kidney stones, treats allergies, asthma

B12 - prevent anaemia, good for concentration, protects nervous system

Vit C - help with absorption of Calcium and iron, enhances immunity, prevents cancer, aids nervous system, proper tissue growth, adrenal gland

Vit D - prevents rickets, normal bone and teeth growth, regulated heartbeat, prevents cancer, enhances immunity

Vit E - antioxidant, prevents cancer and heart disease, prevents cell damage, reduce blood pressure, healthy skin and hair

Vit K - healthy liver function, bone formation, longevity

Calcium - builds healthy bones and teeth, maintains regular heartbeat, stops muscle cramping

Chromium - vital in the making of glucose and metabolism of cholesterol, fats and proteins, maintain blood pressure, maintain blood sugar

Copper - converts iron to haemoglobin, protects against anaemia, healthy bones and joints

Germanium - fight pain, detox the body, enhance immune

Iodine - healthy thyroid gland and metabolize fats

Iron - metabolism, and production of haemoglobin

Magnesium - helps prevent and dissolve kidney stones, helps prevent birth defects, prevents calcification of muscles, improves cardiovascular system, boosts immune, supports and strengthens nervous system

Manganese - needed for healthy nervous system, blood sugar regulation, bone growth, and thyroid hormone production

Selenium - protects immune system, regulates thyroid, supports prostrate gland

Zinc - promotes proper growth, helps with mental clarity and altertness, helps with healing, supports immune

Herbs and Vitamins / Minerals

Alfalfa - vitamin A, B1(Thiamine), Riboflavin, Niacin, B5, B6, B12, C, D, E, K, calcium, iron, magnesium, manganese, selenium, zinc, protein

Aloe Vera - Vitamin A, C, D, B1, B2, germanium, Vitamin E

Burdock root - vitamin A, B1(Thiamine), Riboflavin, Niacin, B5, vit E, C, Calcium, iron, magnesium, manganese, phosphorous, selenium, zinc, folic acid high in potassium, low sodium - blood purifier

Catnip - vitamin B1(thiamine), Riboflavin, Niacin, B6, chromium, iron, magnesium, manganese, selenium,

Cayenne pepper - vitamin A, B1(thiamine), Riboflavin, Niacin, C, calcium, iron, magnesium, selenium, zinc

Chamomile - vitamin B1(thiamine), Riboflavin, Niacin, Calcium, iron, magnesium, manganese, selenium, zinc

Chickweed - vitamin A, B1(thiamine), Riboflavin, Niacin, C, Calcium, iron, magnesium, manganese, potassium, selenium, zinc

Cinnamon - rich with magnesium, good source of iron, and calcium

Comfrey - B12, potassium, sulphur, calcium, iron, phosphorus, Vitamin A, C, B complex, selenium, iron, germanium, protein

Dandelion -high source of vit A & C, high source of vitamin K, vitamin E, high in calcium, folic acid, iron, high in magnesium, manganese, niacin, phosphorus, potassium, riboflavin, zinc

Eyebright - vitamin A, B1(thiamine), Riboflavin, Niacin, C, calcium, iron, magnesium, manganese, zinc

Flaxseed - vitamin E, Calcium, Iron

Garlic - allicin, high source of selenium, rich in potassium, iron, calcium, magnesium, manganese, zinc, vitamin C, B6, tryptophan, phosphorus, B1, copper, protein

Ginger - magnesium, potassium, copper, B6, manganese,

Ginseng - biotin, calcium, copper, choline, germanium, manganese, selenium, zinc, vitamin B Complex, iron

Green Tea - vitamin K, high in antioxidants and alkaloids, Vitamin A, D, E, C, B, B5, H, manganese, zinc, chromium, selenium, very low caffeine content compared to other teas

Hawthorn - selenium, amino acids, calcium, choline, chromium, essential fatty acids, iron, magnesium, manganese, phosphorus, potassium, silicon, zinc, B1, B2, B3, C

Hops - Vitamin A, B1, B2, B3, B6. B12, C, E, calcium, magnesium, manganese, selenium, zinc, phytoestrogens

Lemongrass - vitamin A, calcium, folic acid, iron, magnesium, manganese, selenium, thiamine,

Licorice - Riboflavin, Niacin, chromium, iron, magnesium, amino acids, choline,

Milk Thistle seed - iron, selenium, zinc, silibinin, silymarin,

Mullein - vitamin A, Vitamins B5, B12, D, Choline, Herperidin, sulfur, Riboflavin, Niacin, C, calcium, iron, magnesium, manganese, zinc

Nettles - vitamin A, B1(thiamine), Riboflavin, Niacin, B5, C, D, E, K, calcium, chromium, iron, magnesium, selenium, zinc

Oatstraw - vitamin A, B1(thiamine), Riboflavin, Niacin, B6, C, E, calcium, chromium, iron, magnesium, selenium,

Parsley - Riboflavin, Niacin, Vitamin A, K, C, D, calcium, iron, magnesium, manganese, selenium, zinc, folate

Peppermint - vitamin A, B1(thiamine), Riboflavin, Niacin, C, E, calcium, iron, magnesium, manganese, selenium, potassium,

Plantain - high in potassium, vitamin A, C, calcium, iron,

Raspberry Leaf - vitamin A, B1(thiamine), Riboflavin, Niacin, C, E, calcium, iron, magnesium, manganese, selenium,

Red Clover - vitamin A, B1(thiamine), Riboflavin, Niacin, C, calcium, chromium, magnesium, manganese, molybdenum

Rose Hips - vitamin A, B1(thiamine), Riboflavin, Niacin, C, E, calcium, iron, manganese, selenium, zinc

Rosemary - B complex vitamins, high folates, Vitamin A, Vitamin C, Iron,

Sage - vitamin A, B1(thiamine), Riboflavin, magnesium, zinc, serotonin, rich in B complex, Vitamin C, potassium, manganese, calcium, copper

Yarrow - vitamin B1(thiamine), C, calcium, chromium, magnesium, manganese, selenium,

Yellow Dock - vitamin A, B1(thiamine), beta carotene, Riboflavin, Niacin, B5, C, calcium, high in iron, magnesium, manganese, potassium, selenium

Essential Oils

Essential Oils are an important part of a good home apothecary. You will find them useful in making many home remedies. A few of the most important ones are listed here, with their various possible functions.

Each person who uses essential oils has their own set of favorites. You will find as you start to learn about them, you also will create your own store of favorites in your home that you will use over and over.

- **Carrot Seed oil** - great to help relieve stress and exhaustion, powerful detoxifier and liver booster, rejuvenating to the skin and often used in skin lotions for psoriasis, eczema, carbuncles, boils, etc, fights age
- **Clary Sage** - mild antidepressant, astringent, aphrodisiac, digestive, sedative
- **Eucalyptus** - antibacterial, antimicrobial, antiviral, anti-inflammatory, decongestant, stimulating
- **Grapefruit seed oil** - energizes, brightens dull skin and helps rid toxic build up, helps with reducing water retention, great preservative, antibacterial
- **Lavender** - antibacterial, antimicrobial, antiviral, calms anxiety, blood circulation and respiration
- **Lemon oil** - antibacterial, antimicrobial, antiviral, astringent, detoxifying, energizing, brightens dull skin
- **Orange oil** - antibacterial, anti-inflammatory, diuretic, aphrodisiac, detoxifier, boosts immunity
- **Oregano oil** - antiviral, antibacterial, antimicrobial, really strong oil and will kill most things, never use it straight, always dilute it
- **Peppermint** - indigestion, respiratory problems, headaches, nausea
- **Rosemary** - antibacterial, hair growth, mental activity, respiratory
- **Spearmint** - antibacterial, anti-fungal, insect repellent, restorative, stimulant
- **Tea Tree oil** - antibacterial, antimicrobial, antiviral, insecticide, stimulant, helps with wound healing, detox, relieve pain

Apothecary Essentials

There are a few items that are **extras** that are also needed in a good home apothecary. As we go through some of the remedies, and methods, you will come to understand the importance of each item.

- **Olive oil or jojoba oil** - for salves and moisturizers
- **Coconut oil** - used for so many things, and is so healthy with great antibacterial properties
- **Vodka, vegetable glycerin, apple cider vinegar** - used for making tinctures and glycerites
- **Tea ball, reusable or disposable tea bags** - used for herbal teas and syrups
- **Sugar or honey** - for syrups
- **Beeswax** - for salves and balms to help them solidify
- **Rice, beans, wheat** - for eye and muscle pillows and cold and hot packs

It is always good to try to keep your apothecary items in one location. Dedicate it as your home apothecary spot and keep it well organized and free of other clutter items. You will find that you use it much more frequently when you can easily access what you are looking for. If you don't have a dedicated cupboard or shelve, you can always purchase some plastic drawers. They are fairly inexpensive and you can easily add to them as your apothecary grows. It is a great feeling of accomplishment to have all of your tools and products in one spot and watch it grow and get used often, and with success.

It is always good to have a few good **tools** available for making your home remedies. Following is a good list of tools that will be useful for you as you grow in your apothecary.
- **Capsules and filling tools** - once you learn how easy it is to fill your own capsules, and how inexpensive it is compared to purchasing them in the store, you will do it always
- **strainer / cheesecloth** - to strain herbs from oils and other tinctures and so forth
- **cotton fabric** - for eye and muscle pillows and hot and cold packs
- **jars, tubs, bottles,** and an assortment of these - to store finished products
- **good kitchen scale** - it is important to purchase a good quality kitchen scale. They are not that expensive, and it is well worth it to get a good one. You will use it often

- **Double boiler** - even one that is purchased as a second hand store will be well worth it as you will find in making salves, balms, oils, and a variety of other remedies

- **mortar and pestle** - for grinding up herbs - large herbs into smaller portions

- **labels / felt marker** - always good to make sure everything is labelled and dated properly. You would never want to mix up remedies

- **tea pot** - herbal teas will become a big part of your apothecary so invest in a good tea pot and accessories

- **a variety of sizes of jars** - canning jars of all sizes are great for making tinctures and remedies, you can pick them up cheap at second hand stores, or watch for garage sales as people get rid of them

-**notebook** - to keep in all of your recipes, notes, dates, and all about what you do in one place so you can always refer back to worked great and what didn't

- **library** - a good apothecary will have a library of great books written by those who have already paved the way. No sense in trying to recreate the wheel when it already works. Become an apprentice to a good library of books. They will serve you well.

Preparation Methods

There are several basic ways that herbs can be prepared for use, and they can all easily be prepared right in your own home with a few basic ingredients. Herbal preparations are not a one time cure all process. They are more often taken over longer periods of time, to help bring the body as a whole, into a natural balance. Along with good nutrition and exercise, they will help your body achieve that perfect homoeostasis, or as close to perfect as you can get. Some plants, and some specific parts of plants, work better with certain preparation methods. You will come to understand this better as you work more with herbs.

Some plants and their parts are better used fresh, and others are better dried, ground, made into teas, or compresses, or used in baths. This is because, different techniques are used that are best suited to extract the properties being used, with the least amount of damage and waste.

The most frequently used methods include:
• salves, creams and balms
• teas
• tinctures and glycerites
• syrups
• capsules
• compresses and poultices

Salves, Ointments, and Lotions

One of my all time favorite healing salves is a good calendula salve. A good salve can heal a number of things and calendula salve is definitely one of these.

Salves are easy to make and easy to store. It is made of oils that have been infused - see oil infusion - and then beeswax is added as a hardening agent. These are melted together, and then any other essential oils or other ingredients will be added and mixed well. Then the mixture is poured into containers and allowed to harden.

A standard rule of thumb to follow for the ingredients would be: 2 cups of olive oil infused with your herbs, to 1/2 cup of melted beeswax. If you live in an area that is hotter, you may want to add a bit more beeswax to your recipe. You might have to experiment with this. If you don't have enough added, then you will find you always have a runny, lumpy mess of oil in your containers. There is a way to test it for hardness. If you take a few drops of the oil and beeswax mixture and drop it into a small bowl of really cold water, or put a small spoon of it into the freezer for a short time, you will get a feel for the consistency of the finished product. You should never allow the oil on the stove to come to a boil. Keep it just under that heat. Boiling the oil will kill many of the healing properties that the oil may contain.

A great way to make an all natural petroleum jelly that heals and soothes, is to melt some beeswax into straight olive oil. No infusions or essential oils. Then pour it into containers and allow to harden You could melt it into a coconut oil also, either way it makes a great healing and soothing ointment for chapped skin, or babies bums.

Teas

I am sure that the art of tea making goes back many thousands of years. It is one of the easiest and best ways to get the medicinal properties of herbs into your system in a quick way. A good guide to follow when creating herbal teas is using 1 tablespoon of dried herbs to 1 cup of water. If the herbs are fresh you will want to double that amount. And the standard dose to follow, unless otherwise prescribed, is 1/2 to 1 cup three times a day. There are many different ways to strain your tea, if you aren't using a prepared tea bag. The simplest way would be to purchase a tea ball or tea infuser. There are many available everywhere for fairly inexpensive. And there are some that are much more expensive. You could also use a simple wire sieve or strainer to strain the herbs. It really doesn't matter if there are little bits of the herbs left in the tea, they will carry more nutrients to your body.

There are two ways to make teas, decoctions and infusions.

Decoctions are made by taking an herb, usually a root, berries, or bark part that is tough, and boiling it for several minutes to an hour, to pull the properties out of the herb. It is not really a convenient way to use herbs for first aid because of the length of time it takes. Usually for first aid, these types of herbs will be used as tinctures because they can be already made.

Infusions are like your basic tea. The infusion is usually made with the leaves or flower parts of the herbs as they only need to steep for a while in the boiling water. You simply need to pour boiling water over the herbs and let them steep for a few minutes up to 15 minutes, then pour off the tea and discard the herbs. These can be prepared in larger quantities also and then stored in the fridge to drink cold over a period of a day or two. This is great if you are fighting an illness and you make up a big batch so that you don't have to keep boiling water each time you want to drink a cup of infusion. These can also be used in syrup making, and for compresses.

Poultice and Compress

Compresses and poultices are excellent to use in first aid situations. They get the herbs to the symptom quickly and effectively. A **poultice** consists of herbs that are applied directly to a wound rather than taken internally. For fresh herbs chop them up really fine to mush almost.

For dried herbs you need to make a decoction. For powdered herbs make a paste by mixing with water. Poultice's are normally applied hot, but can also be applied cold. Apply the poultice to the affected area and then cover with a bandage to hold it in place. Replace the poultice every 2 - 4 hours as needed until you get the desired effect.

Compresses can be used on sprains, chest congestion, inflamed areas, sunburns and muscle aches. You simply soak a soft cloth in an herbal infusion and apply with some pressure to the area affected. Re soak the cloth every ½ hour or so and reapply as needed throughout the day and night. Generally a compress is used with a hot water / herb infusion, or tea, but if it is to work on an area that is heat sensitive, then use a cold infusion, however it may take longer to get the specific results. It just depends on what you need.

Oil Infusion

An oil infusion is a process that extracts the medicinal properties out of the plant and captures them into the oils. It is different than essential oils, as they are made by a much more intricate process, and they are pure plant oils. Oil infusions are the medicinal properties in a carrier oil, so weaker than essential oils, however very powerful in their own right and purpose. The carrier oils usually are olive oil, sunflower oil, grape seed oil, but never a cooking oil like canola or corn. Use the purest carrier oil that you can find. It is essential that you always use the best quality of products in all of your medicine making.

Infused oils are used in the process of making massage oils, ointments, salves, balms, creams, and other medicinal remedies. They will usually last at least a year on the shelf if kept in a cool, dark place.

Cold infusion is when you place the herbs in a glass jar and cover with oil of your choice. Stir and shake well, and allow it to sit in a warm sunny spot for four to six weeks. Shake it every day to keep it well mixed up. When time is up strain and squeeze the herbs well, and place the fresh infused oil in a clean jar for use. This is a long slow process, but if you are not in a hurry, it is a great way to create an herbal infused oil. There is also something therapeutic about shaking the herbs, talking to them, and watching them as they create a potent infused oil that will be used to heal.

Hot oil infusion is a much quicker way get the end product. You prepare the herbs and oil just the same as you would with the cold infusion, but place your glass jar in a pot of water on the stove, or in a crock pot that has a couple of inches of water in the bottom, on lowest setting. You don't want to bring the oil to a boil, but let it steep on low heat for several hours or up to 3 days. Make sure you add water as it evaporates. If you are worried that the jar might break, you can place a small towel on the bottom of the pot in the water. I have also placed the herbs and oil strait into the top of a double boiler and let them heat on low for an hour or two. This is the quickest method if you are in a hurry, but again be careful not to let the oil come to a boil. The herbs will be crispy when you go to strain them out, but that is what they are supposed to be like.

Tinctures, Glycerites and Vinegars

These are really easy to prepare, but take time to process. Tinctures are usually prepared with some form of alcohol, like vodka, that is strong and pure. The more pure the better. Alcohol is a great preservative, and also pulls out the medicinal properties of the herbs. Glycerites are made using 100% vegetable glycerin instead of alcohol. This is great for those who are alcohol intolerant, or children. I personally am not a fan of alcohol, and prefer to use glycerin. It is important to know the properties of the herb that you want to be tincturing because some of them are not soluble in glycerin, only alcohol. Sometimes apple cider vinegar can replace the alcohol. This is why it is important to know your herb.

Tincturing is simple. You place the desired herb or herbs, into a glass jar. Make sure they are chopped up small. Cover the herbs with the alcohol, glycerin, vinegar, or combination. Let sit and brew for several weeks. Shake daily. Strain well when done and squeeze out all the liquid from the herbs. Voila! That is all there is to it. Depending on which menstruum you use, your tincture will have a pretty long shelf life if kept out of the sun and heat.

Vodka is often used as an excellent medium for extracting the medicinal properties. An alcohol based tincture has a near indefinite shelf life, just sitting there looking pretty. Alcohol is actually is better than glycerin or vinegar because both of those don't extract all of the properties, just most of them. Alcohol based tinctures are highly concentrated and you don't have to use much at all of the finished product to get the desired results. A typical dose of a tincture like this is about 1 tbsp added to a cup of juice or water. This can be taken 2 or 3 times per day as needed, or more for an acute problem. However for those that are alcohol intolerant, pregnant, recovering alcoholics, or children, it is best to use a vegetable glycerin mixture with water, or a vinegar such as apple cider vinegar. Regular white vinegar is not good to use for this process. Alcohol based tinctures are also great for wounds. They have super antibacterial properties and can kill the bacteria that may be present in a wound. The alcohol is a great disinfectant and the herbs are great everything else. If you are alcohol intolerant for some reason, then adding the tsp or tbsp to a cup of hot water or juice will evaporate the alcohol within a few minutes, then you can consume it without any worry.

Some recipes for tincture making will give you a ratio for the measurements. This, for example, 1:5 would mean that you would use 1 part herb to 5 parts alcohol. Take note from the recipes also whether the recipe is written in weighted measurements, or measuring cup measurements. It makes a difference to know which you are using.

Glycerites are often called syrups because the glycerin is so sweet. However it is the exact same process as tincturing with alcohol, except your medium would be made up of approximately 75% vegetable glycerin, and 25% distilled or purified water. Then the process is the same as if you were using an alcohol like vodka. These are great for pregnant ladies, children, and people who are intolerant to alcohol. They don't have quite as long of a shelf life as an alcohol tincture, but their shelf life is still a couple of years or more.

Syrups are made other ways than a tincture. If you make a strong tea out of the herbs you want to use, and then add honey or sugar that is all there is to making a syrup. The normal amount of sugar or honey to add is one cup per 2 cups of liquid. Heat it all so it is dissolved and mixed well together. Remember doing this, you don't want to bring honey to a boil because it will destroy any of its healing properties. If you are using sugar, then you can boil the concoction down to the desired thickness. You only need it to be slightly thicker than the infusion, reason being, so it will linger or coat the lining of the throat. This will help allow the properties to get to work quickly and in the right spots. Once done, pour it into a bottle, label it well and refrigerate it. Use as needed. Most of these syrups need to be refrigerated to preserve them long.

Vinegars, specifically apple cider vinegar, is a great medium as well to extract the medicinal properties, but it isn't as potent as an alcohol based tincture. It also doesn't have as long of a shelf life. They are a good alternative if you can't take the alcohol, because they are similar in which properties they will extract that perhaps the glycerin's won't.

Capsules

I love making my own herbal capsules. The first time I did this I was amazed at how little herb goes into each capsule. To purchase herbs bulk, and then capsule them yourself, saves a whole lot of money. The most expensive part is purchasing the capsules themselves. You will also need to purchase a capsule machine. You can purchase the capsule machine and gel caps for fairly inexpensive from The Bulk Herb Store online. Gel caps come in different sizes so depending on if you have problems swallowing larger capsules then you will want the small "O" size. But if you want to get more herb into you, then purchase the "OO" size. Gel caps also come in vegetarian gel caps and non vegetarian, depending on your preference. Making your own capsules also will guarantee that you know what is going into your capsules, and how fresh the herbs are. If you can grow your own herbs, even better because then you know exactly how fresh they are, and you don't have to buy them!

Labelling

First off, before you get started creating all kinds of salves and remedies, it is important to know how to properly label everything. There are a few things that should be on your labels. The date the item was made, the ingredients in it, and how to use it are the most important. If you don't put on the label how to use the item, then it may sit there in your kit and never get used. If your family doesn't know how to use it, and it isn't on the label, it is likely it won't get used. Don't assume that others will know anything, because they won't!

Always date it so you can be aware of possible expiry dates. If something is starting to smell a bit off, then you can check the date to see how old it is. Dating it is very important because rancid oils, salves, or tinctures can make you pretty sick, and they smell nasty too. Most things have a pretty long shelf life, but nevertheless don't trust to that. Another reason to date your items, so when you know that something worked really well and you are almost out of it, you can check the date, and then check back into your journal or record book to see for sure the recipe and any notes you may have made while making the recipe. If something works, you don't want to have to reinvent the wheel or search all over for the information to make it again. Record it in your journal and date everything.

It is important to have the ingredients on the label also. Many people have different allergies and you don't know what they are, so make it visible for people to see what they are using. Some ingredients might affect others differently, so they will know to watch out for them. For example cayenne pepper must not be used by children, that should be on the label. Don't assume people know! They don't!

Remedies and Recipes

You can heal yourself and your family by making remedies in your own kitchen. They are much cheaper, and more importantly, they are much healthier than the drugstore alternatives. Making your own remedies isn't hard, and once you understand the processes involved, it will become second nature to you to just whip up whatever concoction it is that you need. This small recipe section will give you a good assortment of basic things that can be created in your own home apothecary. Of course, you should always be doing your own research too, as there are many other things that can be created like: soap, shampoo bars, all kinds of teas, tinctures, and so many more remedies. This is just a basic sampler for you, with some of the best remedies I have found.

Pain Relief and Healing

Tension Headache Infusion

1 part skullcap

1 part sage

1 part peppermint

1/4 part lavender

Mix the herbs well. When you feel a headache coming on, use 2 tsp in one cup of boiling water for 10 - 15 minutes. Add honey or lemon and drink as much as you need to get your desired effects.

Arnica oil

Olive oil infused with dried arnica flowers. Prepare infusion and bottle and label well. This can be stored for up to a year or longer. **Arnica is one of the best pain reliever**s for sprains and sore muscles. Apply to bruises and sore muscles for fast relief and reduce swelling. Don't use on broken skin.. Label well. **Arnica is not to be taken internally.**

Deep Heat Muscle Rub

Make a salve using the following herbs infused into olive oil and hardened with beeswax.

16 ounces wintergreen essential oil

3 parts St. John's wort

3 parts skullcap

1 part cayenne pepper

This can also be used as an oil rub, just eliminate the beeswax and use it as a massage oil. But when using as an oil, be careful it will stay on your hands and the cayenne can burn when rubbed into eyes or nose or face.

Migraine Tincture

3 parts lemon balm

3 parts feverfew

2 parts valerian root

1 part St. John's wort

100 proof vodka or 60% glycerin and 40% water to fill jar tincture for 2 -6 weeks. Strain, bottle and store for up to 5 years. At the first signs of a migraine take ½ tsp every 30 minutes to an hour until symptoms subside.

Lobelia Tincture or Capsules

Lobelia is often used as a migraine or headache relief. It can be used as a tincture or in capsule form. Follow the instructions carefully because if over used it can cause nausea and vomiting. But used in moderation it is great for relieving headaches. For more chronic headaches a person should dig to the root of the problem and treat with herbs accordingly.

Valerian Tincture

Valerian is one of stinkiest herbs I have ever smelled. But boy does it work. It has great antispasmodic properties and is a great painkiller too. It will relieve intestinal and cramps associated with women's cycles. It is great for headaches, general aches, pains, and will bring on sleep when nothing else will.

2 parts valerian root

½ part hop flowers

100 proof vodka or 60% glycerin and 40% water

Tincture for 2 - 6 weeks shaking daily. Strain well. Store in clean jar in dark place. It will keep for up to five years.

Stress Relief Formula

Make a tincture or glycerite from the following.

2 parts valerian root

1 part each: passionflower, hops flowers, skullcap, wild yam. Can be used for adults or children. Good to use for tension and muscle spasm, insomnia, relaxation, anxiety and panic.

Restless Leg Syndrome Salve

1 part devils club

1 part skullcap

1 part chamomile

Infuse some olive oil or your favorite other oil, I actually use the Balm of Gilead oil before it is made into a salve and infuse these herbs into this oil. Once they have been infused, strain the oil well and add beeswax following the standard of about 1/4 cup grated beeswax per 1 cup of infused oil. Melt beeswax and pour into sterile containers.

Vapour Rub

4 ounces of olive oil melted with ½ ounce of beeswax

Add 2 tsp eucalyptus oil

2 tsp peppermint oil

2 tsp thyme oil

Pour into containers and let harden. Use for nasal congestion and common cold symptoms. Use for flu, coughs on chest, and sinus headaches. It is great to rub on chest, back, feet, under nose and on your temples. It does a great job of opening up the sinus.

Cold and Flu Tincture or Glycerite

2 ounces dried echinacea root

1 ounce goldenseal

1 ounce elderberries

1 ounce dried lemon balm

1 ounce dried horehound

vodka or a mix of 60% vegetable glycerin and 40% water, enough to fill a jar

Steep in jar for 2 - 6 weeks, shaking daily. Vodka tincture will be good for 5 years on the shelf. The glycerite will be about half that shelf life. Adults as sign of colds ¼ - ½ tsp every 30 minutes to hour until symptoms subside.

Cold Capsules

1 part echinacea root powder

1 part rose hips powder

1 part goldenseal powder

¼ part cayenne pepper powder

Mix well and make capsules using capsule machine. At first sign of being sick take 1 - 2 capsules every 2 - 3 hours. Continue for 2 days then reduce dosage to 6 capsules a day until better.

Immune Boost Formula - there are many different formulas that will boost your immunity. Use this formula to make a tincture with vodka or glycerin and water, depending on if you are alcohol intolerant or making it for children.

9 parts echinacea root

3 parts goldenseal

1 part each: siberian ginseng root, usnea, fresh garlic

For maintenance you could use a couple of dropperfuls each day. Then at first signs of illness up this to 1 - 2 dropperfuls every hour until symptoms stop.

Elderberry syrup

1 cup of dried elderberries

3 cups water

1 cup honey

2 tbsp grated ginger root - optional

Simmer berries and ginger in water over low heat for 45 minutes. Smash the berries well. Strain through a cheesecloth. Add honey and stir well. Bottle syrup and store in fridge for up to 3 months. Use as needed for coughs and colds. Great immune booster. 1 tsp per day for prevention for children. 1 tsp per hour at first signs of cold and flu. Adults 1 tbsp.

Elderberry glycerite

1 cup vegetable glycerin

1 cup water

½ pound dried berries

in quart jar place dried elderberries. Mix the glycerin and water together and pour over berries. Shake daily for 4 - 6 weeks. Strain well squeezing well. Store in an airtight container for up to six months on the shelf. Good and safe for pregnant mothers and infants. 1 tsp daily for prevention and 4 tsp daily at first signs of illness.

Comfrey Calendula Salve

1 ¼ c olive oil

equal parts of comfrey, calendula, and st john's wort

1 - 2 ounces beeswax

Infuse the herbs into the oil. Make salve with the oil. This is a great healing salve for small cuts, bruises and so forth. It is not good for deep cuts because of the comfrey. Comfrey will heal the outside of the wound too quickly and often the deep tissue isn't healed and infection can occur. Comfrey is great for broken bones and helping them heal. It is great for minor cuts and scrapes, but not deep cuts. This is also a great healing salve for burns and rashes and bites.

Neosporin

1 ½ ounces beeswax grated

1 cup olive oil, almond, or coconut oil. To add some extra healing, infuse your oil with calendula petals

¼ tsp vitamin E oil

½ tsp tea tree oil

20 drops lavender essential oil

10 drops lemon essential oil

Melt oils and beeswax over low heat. Remove from heat and add vitamin E oil and essential oils. Stir well. Pour into small jars or containers. Use as you would a neosporin or polysporin or antiseptic ointment.

Kloss's Herbal Liniment a great ointment very popular and recipe readily available in most herb books and web sites.

1 ounce echinacea powder

1 ounce goldenseal root powder

2 ounces myrrh gum powder

½ ounce cayenne pepper powder

rubbing alcohol to cover - approximately 1 quart

Place herbs in a clean glass jar. Fill with rubbing alcohol leaving an inch head space. Mix and blend well. Let stand in a warm spot for about 4 weeks. This is different from a tincture because it is only to be used externally. Make sure it is clearly labelled this way. After it has steeped for 4 weeks, strain well and re-bottle. Label well. This liniment can be applied every few minutes for an hour or two in acute instances. Use freely until desired results. If bottled in spray bottles it is really easy to use. This liniment is so powerful it will stop a stye from developing on the eye by dabbing on with a q tip. Don't get in eye. By applying to temples, back of neck, and to forehead it can e used as an excellent remedy for a headache. Spray on swollen joints or arthritis spots for relief. Can also be used on cuts, ringworm, sprains, sunburn, poison ivy, and chicken pox.

Drawing Salve - Black salve

Can be applied to boils, stings, bites, slivers, and anything that needs to draw out infection or object. These measurements are weighted measurements, not amounts. Use your kitchen scale to weigh them.

6 ounces of olive oil infused with goldenseal, chickweed, and plantain equal parts of each

2 ounces castor oil - it has great drawing properties

1 ounce beeswax grated

½ cup activated charcoal

½ c bentonite clay

1 tsp of each essential oil, clove, rosemary, lemon, lavender, and eucalyptus

Infuse oil over the stove with the herbs for a couple of hours. Strain well and return to stove on low heat. Stir in beeswax until melted. Remove from heat and stir in castor oil, charcoal, clay, and essential oils. Stir and mix well. Pour into a glass jar or tins and label well. Store in a cool dark place. Place small amount of salve to affected area and keep bandaged for 12 hours, redoing every 2 hours until healed. This stuff is amazing to suck out pretty much anything.

Activated Charcoal for drawing poultice

Activated charcoal is great if you don't have the Black Salve. Simply make a paste out of the charcoal and some water and paste it onto the sting, sliver, or infection and wrap it well with clean gauze or cloth. Replace often, like every couple of hours, until you get the desired results. It can draw out poisons from an insect bite like spiders, bees or wasps. Be careful though on applying it to open wounds, as it can leave a good tatoo scar.

Activated charcoal is used to treat poisoning, and help with intestinal gas, lower cholesterol, and even help prevent hangovers. It is the best antidote for poisoning bar none, and it can save your life. It does this because it is the best at capturing chemicals and prevents their absorption into your system. Get capsules into your system as quickly as possible for poisoning.

It is great taken internally to help absorb the toxins, acids, heavy metals, and other things that can build up in the system. Simply take the charcoal until the symptoms disappear. There is no danger of overdosing on charcoal. The only recommendation is to take lots of water to help flush your system and prevent constipation.

For other problems, use as needed to help you feel better, but follow directions on the bottle if you have purchased capsules. It would be important to use capsules for these purposes, so either purchase some capsules, or make your own capsules and have them readily available for anytime use. Always carry activated charcoal with you in your herbal first aid kit. It is safe to use on anyone.

Balm of Gilead Salve

You need to find a nice grove of poplar trees, because the "Balm of Gilead" is the resin on the buds of the poplar tree. Any type of poplar tree will do, it doesn't have to be a specific variety. Very first thing in the spring as the tree is starting to bud out, you will notice that the buds have a very sticky resin that oozes from them. This is the prime time to pick the buds. A cool day would be best because the buds aren't quite as sticky, but any time will do. Harvest yourself a cup or two of the nice swollen resinous buds. Pick a few off each branch, so you don't stress out any one particular branch of the tree. Once you have a nice stash, add them to a jar and cover them with olive oil with a couple of inches to spare, because they will swell a bit more in the oil. Let them sit in the oil for a couple of weeks up to 2 months to let the oil absorb as much of the resin as possible. Shake it well everyday because the resin will settle to the bottom of the jar. When it is done soaking, strain it out well and gently heat the oil over a low burner. Add about 1/4 cup of grated beeswax to each cup of oil that you end up with. When it is all melted, pour into clean sterile containers and allow to harden. ** You could add some carrot seed oil to this salve - it is great for psoriasis and eczema and most skin problems. Balm of Gilead salve is also great for muscle aches and joint pains. It tends to drive deep into muscles, so can be used for any deep tissue salve.

Calendula Salve or Miracle Balm

This can either be poured into small tins, jars, or push up containers.

1 ¼ c olive oil

1/3 ounce of dried calendula flowers

1/3 ounce dried plantain

¼ ounce dried St. John's Wort

¼ ounce dried Oregon grape root

1 - 2 ounces beeswax - I tend to add the greater amount so the salve doesn't melt in hot weather

Essential oils to add might be lemon, eucalyptus, lemongrass, and lavender. These all have some great healing properties, as well as great preservative properties for the salve to last longer. Infuse the herbs into the oil using the hot oil method mentioned earlier. When done strain the herbs out well. Return the oil to the pot and add the beeswax. Melt over low heat.

Remove from heat and add any essential oils you might want to add. Remember with essential oils, a little goes a long way. When stirred in, pour into clean sterile containers. Allow to harden. Place on lid and label well.

Plantain Bite and Sting Poultice

fresh plantain leaves

I love **plantain**. It is as common almost as **dandelion** once you know what you are looking for. Pick some fresh plantain leaves and mash well making a poultice. You could also chew them well and apply directly to wound for immediate relief of bite or sting. It is also great for small cuts, rashes, bruises, and almost anything minor if you are outside not close to anything else.

Itch relief stick

1 ounce of olive oil (more if needed to cover herbs completely) infused with calendula flowers, chickweed, nettle leaf, lemon balm leaf, plantain leaf about 2 tbsp of each

1 ounce shea butter 2 tbsp or coconut oil will work also

1 ounce or more of beeswax 2 - 4 tbsp

2 tsp essential oil blend of citronella oil, lavender oil, rosemary oil, tea tree oil

Melt all the oils, except essential oils, and butters together over low heat. Add grated beeswax and melt. Remove from heat and stir in essential oils. Stir in well and pour into a empty push up container. Use as needed for bites and rashes.

Bug repellant spray

1 ounce rubbing alcohol or witch hazel

1 ounce grape seed oil or olive oil

30 drops citronella essential oil

20 drops eucalyptus essential oil, this could be substituted with tea tree oil

15 drops lemon or lemongrass or a combination essential oil

15 drops cedar essential oils

Mix well in a spray bottle and use when outdoors. Spray again every couple of hours as needed.

Dandelion leaf tea

It is easy to make and super nourishing. Pick some fresh leaves. Let them dry. And make a tea infusion with them. A dandelion leaf tea is a great way to flush any excess water from your system. It is a great diuretic and also contains vitamin A, calcium, potassium and other vitamins and minerals. All in all it is a very nutritious tonic / tea to drink or eat in salads every day.

Varicose Vein Rub

Fill a quart jar with half and half dried calendula flowers and dried yarrow leaves and flowers. You could add in another part of lavender buds if you have them on hand, and then reduce the amount of lavender essential oil that you add in at the end. Cover the mix of dried herbs with witch hazel and allow it to sit for about 3 - 4 weeks, shaking it daily to mix it well. Strain out the herbs and discard them. Add in 25 drops of lavender oil. Mix well. Pour into a spray bottle, or another container. Label it well. This can be sprayed or rubbed on the varicose veins as often as you want.

The calendula helps to strengthen the capillary and vein walls. It is also anti-inflammatory. The yarrow will help to get blood circulation going properly, which helps with removing any blood that may have been pooling in the veins. The lavender has great healing properties and will help stop the itching that is often associated with varicose veins. The witch hazel is a strong astringent and will help to shrink the enlarged veins and tissue surrounding them.

Body Care

Basic Lip Balm

3 tsp beeswax

2 tsp coconut oil

1 vitamin E capsule

2 - 3 drops favorite flavor essential oil

Melt coconut oil and beeswax. Remove from heat. Add vitamin E and essential oil flavoring when slightly cooled. If it is too hot, it will evaporate some of the essential oils. Pour into lip tubes and let set. Use your creativity and experiment with different flavors, you can find some great ones.

Chocolate Mint Lip Balm

Using the basic lip balm recipe, add into the melting oils 3 tbsp dark cocoa. When adding in the essential oils, use peppermint oil. It will make a delicious flavoured chocolate mint lip balm.

Basic Lip Balm #2 - makes 4 - 1 oz tins

7 tsp grated beeswax

6 tsp coconut oil

6 tsp jojoba oil

1 1/2 tsp vitamin E oil

1 tsp essential oils or more

Melt everything together except the essential oils. When slightly cooled, pour in essential oils. Pour into tins or tubes and let set.

Imitation Burt's Bees Lip Balm - makes about 40 small tubes

Melt 4 oz of beeswax on low heat.

Add: 3 oz coconut oil

1 oz pure Shea butter

Stir on low heat until all melted. Drop in 30 drops of peppermint oil or slightly more, and 20 drops rosemary oil. Fill tubes. It will cool quickly, so pour quickly.

Basic Solid Perfume Base

3 parts fixed oil - almond or jojoba or coconut

3 parts beeswax grated

1 part fragrance essential oils: patchouli, rose, jasmine, etc.

Melt oil and wax on low. Remove from heat and add in essential oils. Pour into containers quickly and allow to harden.

Rain smell: 5 drops sandalwood, 10 drops bergamot, 10 drops cassia

Jasmine and Lavender are a nice blend

A "dirty hippie" blend includes: patchouli, lemongrass, cedarwood, sweet orange, clary sage, lavender, and pine

Basic Aftershave

Helps to open the pores and soften facial hair so it is easier to shave.

1 cup of witch hazel extract

10 drops of orange essential oil or the zest of one orange

10 drops of cinnamon oil or one cinnamon stick

5 drops clove oil or 3 clove buds

5 drops allspice oil

1 tsp glycerin

1 tsp aloe vera gel - optional

pint jar

Mix all together in a jar and place lid on it. Shake well and shake every day for 4 - 6 weeks.

When done, strain off ingredients and place in a dark bottle. Use as needed after shaving.

Basic Hand and Body Cream

This doesn't leave a greasy feeling. It is great for dry skin.

1/3 cup Extra Virgin Olive Oil

1 tbps aloe vera gel

2 tbsp coconut oil

1 tbsp beeswax

4 tbsp hydrosol

essential oils according to smell or healing properties

Mix together olive oil and aloe vera gel. Set aside. Melt coconut oil and beeswax. Add the olive oil and aloe to mixture. Add hydrosol while blending in processor until smooth. Transfer to jars and let cool.

Delicious Herbal Recipes

Dandelion coffee - caffeine free

If you love coffee but can't handle the caffeine, or just want a healthier choice, try dandelion coffee. It is really quite delicious. Chop up some fresh roots. Place them into a nicely seasoned cast iron pan, and roast them until they have turned a nice dark brown and have a nice fragrance of roasted coffee. Use about 2 tsp to 1 cup of water and simmer for 10 minutes. Strain and enjoy. Add honey or milk as desired for flavor. Dandelion root is a great liver tonic. It will help your liver function top notch and help remove any toxins.

Dandelion Garlic Pesto

3 cloves of garlic crushed

1/2 cup olive oil

2 cups fresh young dandelion leaves - this can be substituted with chickweed or nettles both are also highly nutritious

1/4 cup Parmesan cheese - fresh grated is the best

sea salt to taste

lemon juice or lime juice to taste

Place garlic, oil and leaves in blender. blend well. It should be a little runny. Place in a bowl and add the remaining ingredients. Mix well. Use as a dip with crackers, or bread. Use on pasta or fish or whatever you think it will taste good with.

Sauteed Dandelion Roots

Pick, wash and chop up some dandelion roots. Fresh in the spring is best, but they can be used throughout the growing season. In a fry pan, heat: 2 tbsp sesame oil, 3 tbsp soy sauce, and a small amount of rice vinegar. Add 1 cup of chopped onion and a couple of garlic cloves chopped small. Saute these until they are translucent. Add in about 2 cups of the dandelion roots cut and saute for about 10 minutes until the roots are tender.

Dandelion Chai - caffeine free

1 part dried dandelion root

1 part dried dandelion leaf

1/8 part crushed cardamom

1/8 part crushed cloves

1/8 part crushed cinnamon sticks

1/8 part dried ginger pieces

1/8 part allspice

1/16 - 1/8 part peppercorns whole

1 vanilla bean crushed

Use approximately 1 tbsp of mixture per cup of boiling water. Cover and let steep for about 10 minutes. Strain the herbs from the tea. Add milk and honey according to your tastes. Serve hot.

Herbal Chai - caffeine free

4 cups boiling water

2 cinnamon sticks

1 tbsp grated ginger

1 tbsp cardamom

1 tsp clove buds

1/2 tsp peppercorns

1/2 tsp anise seeds

Simmer these in the boiling water for about 15 minutes. You can add in a black or green tea if you want. Add these in to the hot water after the herbs are finished boiling and strained, then allow to steep for a few minutes. Or add in 1/2 tsp echinacea root and 1/2 tsp astragalus root for an added boost of health. Add honey or warm milk to taste as you like.

Sweet and Spicy Tea

1/2 cup dried balm

1/2 cup chamomile flowers

1/4 cup dried orange mint / or chocolate mint

1/4 cup dried grated orange peel

1/2 tbsp whole cloves

1/2 cinnamon stick crushed

1 tbsp dried stevia leaves

Mix all ingredients well and store in an airtight jar. Use approximately 1 tsp - 1 tbsp per cup of boiling water. Pour over herbs and allow to steep for a few minutes. Strain and serve hot or chilled on a hot day.

Nutritious Herbal Vinegars

This is packed full with nutrition. Fill a jar full with herbs from the list below, or add your own according to your tastes. Then cover it with apple cider vinegar and place a lid on it. Label it well and let sit for six weeks as you shake it daily. After the six weeks, strain off the vinegar and discard the herbs. Use the vinegar over your favorite salad or as a dip with breads.

Herbs you could use:

Alfalfa leaves

Chamomile flowers

Calendula petals

Dandelion leaves and/or roots

Nettle leaves

Hawthorn berries

Burdock roots

Cleavers leaves

Chickweed leaves

Cayenne pepper

Stinging Nettle - can be substituted in any recipe that you would use spinach and it is very nutritious. It tastes similar as well. Great to pick fresh and use as spinach, however pick it using gloves because it can cause your skin to hurt and develop quite a rash.

Rose Hip Honey

Gather the rose hips, just before or after the first frost. They are actually best just after a frost. Freeze the rose hips in a baggie in your freezer. When they are frozen remove the seeds and fill a glass jar with the pulp from the rose hips. Fill the jar with honey and stir it well. Let it sit on the counter for at least three days. You can shake your jar daily or turn it over just to keep things mixed up well. You can now use it on toast or in teas. It is great, and packed full of vitamin C, and potassium. This doesn't need to be stored in the fridge unless you need to keep it for long term.

Hawthorn Honey

Fill a jar with nice ripe berries. If you only have dried berries, you can rehydrate them, drain of any excess liquid, or drink it, and then fill the jar with the re hydrated berries. Cover them with honey and stir well. Let is sit, stirring or turning daily, for 3 days to 3 weeks. Use as honey on toast, or in teas, or however you like. If you need to keep it for longer term, then it will keep best in the fridge.

Burdock Root

Burdock Root can be used in any stir fry recipe, soups, and in your teas. To use in stir fries, wash, cut and add to your other vegetable. Burdock can be a bit gaseous, so mix well with other vegetables, don't make a meal just out of the root. Use the same with soups or stew, wash and cut similar to a carrot or turnip and add to your soup. It is highly nutritious.

Elderberry Syrup

If you have fresh berries, they are the best, but if not use dried ones and place them in a pot with just enough water to cover the berries. Simmer them until they begin to be kind of mush. You can help them by using a utensil to smash them as they cook. Cook well enough to get all the juice out of the berries. When they are done, strain the berries through a cheesecloth or similar type cloth. Squeeze them well to get all the juice out of them. While the juice is still warm, add some honey, usually an equal amount as the liquid. Stir it in and mix it well. You can reheat it a little just to melt the honey if you need to. Bottle it up and store it in the fridge. It is a great immune booster and tastes great too.

Herbal Jellos

Depending on which herbs you are wanting to get into your children or fussy adults, especially when they are sick, create your herb jello by first starting off with your tea. Whichever herbs you want, create your tea with them. For 1 box of jello, use 1 cup of the prepared herbal tea, hot.

Mix this in with the jello powder and stir until the powder is dissolved. When the powder is dissolved, add in 1 cup of cold herbal tea. Stir well and allow to set in the refrigerator. If you want more of a finger jello texture, then add half the amount of cold tea at the end instead of the full cup. Feed the little ones, or the big ones, the jello as they will eat it, when sick. This can also be drank as a warm drink for upset tummies after the cold tea is added, before it is refrigerated and set. That is always a favorite of my children.

Powerhouse Seasoning

Highly nutritious, highly antioxidant, high in fatty acids, what more could you want? Oh ya, tastes great too! Use on salads, vegetables, meat, grains, legumes, and pretty much everything to give you a boost and great taste.

equal parts dried herbs: nettle leaf, dandelion leaf, plantain leaf, thyme leaf, parsley leaf, sage leaf, oregano leaf, alfalfa leaf, cayenne pepper (half part or less according to tastes), chickweed, and chopped dried garlic or garlic powder (half part according to tastes).

Measure all herbs and place in a glass jar. Mix it very well. Store in an empty spice jar and fill as needed. If it is in an empty spice jar kept handy, you will use it more often. It should stay fresh for up to a year if kept out of light and away from heat. Other herbs you might want to add: tarragon, rosemary, fennel, dill, chives, basil, yarrow leaves. This would also make an excellent gift.

Green Herbal Smoothie Mix or Green Juice
Equal Parts of each dried herb: spirulina, nettle leaf, alfalfa leaf, rose hips, marshmallow root, slippery elm bark, raspberry leaf, dandelion leaf, plantain leaf, chickweed

Mix all herbs together in a blender. Pulse until the herbs are chopped very fine, as close to powder as possible. Store in an airtight container. Add 1 tsp of powder to smoothie or fresh juice each day. You could add it to water with a little lemon or lime juice also. Mix well and drink cold. It is a great nutritional drink. You own homemade green juice

Herbal First Aid

We are living in a world where we can't rely on our health care systems to always provide what we need, and as a society we depend way to much on running to the hospital for every little sniffle or ache. It all costs money, and usually ends up in some prescription drug being pushed through our body. Have we lost the ability to care for ourselves in this system? It seems that the "doctor" is the only one who knows best, and in some cases this is definitely true, however, for many things, we can easily treat ourselves and loved ones, if we just knew a few things about plants and what to do with them.

I love to be outdoors. My family loves to camp and be outdoors, in the mountains. It makes sense that we carry with us an herbal first aid kit, and learn what to do with the plants that we come across in nature.

This portion of this book has been written and compiled as I have researched the best remedies and helps that I could find, to put together my own pretty inclusive herbal first aid kit. My kits are always improving as I learn more, but I feel that with what I have gathered, and shared here, I could pretty much cover any minor, and a few major, illnesses or injuries that the average family might come across.

Of course, please also do your own research since there are always new and improved ideas. But, in doing this remember, we don't have to reinvent the wheel. Use the information that others have already found to be tried and true.

When I was on the hunt of how to put together an herbal first aid kit, I did a lot of research, to try and figure out just what was the best way to go about doing this. I found so much information out there in cyber-world, and in books upon books. It was almost overwhelming. I just wanted someone to tell me, here is what you should have, and here is how you should make it. Well I realized that there is just no one perfect form of an herbal first aid kit, because everyone loves different herbs for different uses. I decided that I would put together my own basic kit, with the recipes that I love, and make it so others looking for a simple kit, could follow what I have come up with.

One of the things that I learned, was to study the local herbs that are abundant in my area, find out everything they are good for, and use them. This will save you money, and will always ensure a plentiful supply of medicine. If they don't grow locally, then perhaps you could purchase seeds and grow them yourself. There is a great satisfaction in growing your own herbs, harvesting and making medicine with them.

Out of this quest to develop my own basic herbal first aid kit, developed this portion of Bitter Sweet Herbals. Experiment with each of the remedies that are listed here and adjust to your own liking. Then when you have learned what each one does, you can add it to your first aid kit with the confidence that you will know how to use it when the need arises.

Always keep a Quick Reference Guide for ailments, with your first aid kit. It may be you that is in need of first aid and someone else will have to figure out what to use. A quick reference guide will be essential, for often, if we are experiencing one of our children or a loved one with an injury or ailment, we are not always able to think straight. Have your quick reference guide memorized and accessible so it will be easy to know what products to use for what injury.

There are a few things that should be in every well rounded herbal first aid kit. We will take some time now to go over each of them. It is important to know that this book isn't meant to be a way to self diagnose your symptoms. It really is meant to help treat first aid issues. If you have medical emergencies, serious injuries, or and kind of chronic conditions, you really should seek medical attention. Make sure that when you are learning to use herbs, you are aware of their properties, to help prevent any unwanted concerns. For example, some herbs should not be used if pregnant, be aware of these cautions, some are stimulants, some are astringent, and so forth. If you know what the herb's actions are, then you will quickly be able to respond and know which herb to use for which ailment. I have discussed this a bit already in the first portion of the book.

To Label or Not to Label

First off, before you get started creating all kinds of salves and remedies, it is important to know how to properly label everything. There are a few things that should be on your labels. The date the item was made, the ingredients in it, and how to use it are the most important. If your family doesn't know how to use it, and it isn't on the label, it won't get used. Don't assume that others will know anything, because they won't!

Always date it so you can be aware of possible expiry dates. If something is starting to smell a bit off, then you can check the date to see how old it is. Dating it is very important because rancid oils, salves, or tinctures can make you pretty sick, and they smell nasty too. Most things have a pretty long shelf life, but nevertheless don't trust to that. Another reason to date your items, so when you know that something worked really well and you are almost out of it, you can check the date, and then check back into your journal or record book to see for sure the recipe and any notes you may have made while making the recipe. If something works, you don't want to have to reinvent the wheel or search all over for the information to make it again. Record it in your journal and date everything.

It is important to have the ingredients on the label also. Many people have different allergies and you don't know what they are, so make it visible for people to see what they are using. Some ingredients might affect others differently, so they will know to watch out for them. For example cayenne pepper must not be used by children, that should be on the label. Don't assume people know! They don't!

I keep a record book of each item I make, whether it is a tincture, salve, balm, or tea. My book is just a regular notebook, and I record in it the date of the item made, what was in it, and how I made it. If I made it for a particular person, I will write that in my notes. If I use homegrown herbs or home made items, I will put that in my notes. Basically I journal entry the details of making each remedy. I want to know if it worked well, or not, and also I will go back and record the results or response of how it worked, or didn't.

Kits

I actually have two herbal first aid kits and am in need of a third one, or two bigger ones. My kits are actually tool kits, and I use these for a couple of reasons. One, they are really strong and durable with lots of compartments. Two, they are easy to carry and transport when I go somewhere. These kits come in all shapes and sizes so you can be creative with how you want to put together your kit.

My smaller kit contains all of my essential oils and some quick reference guides on some of the more important oils that get used for many things, like Tea Tree oil and Oregano oil. My bigger kit contains my salves, a few tinctures, bandages, dried herbs, and a lot of the different remedies, teas, salves, and things that I have listed here. It is bulging at the seams though, and I am in need of another kit, and then to sort and organize a bit more. This seems to be an ongoing process as I add to it.

It is important that not only you can find things quickly in your kits, but that your whole family is able to find what they need and use what they find. Perhaps even taking time to teach your family at least a few of the basic most important items that are found in the kit, and how to use them, will be beneficial when the time for first aid arrives.

Quick Reference Guide for First Aid

- **Acid Reflux** - drink a cup of marshmallow tea or take two capsules with water. Do this as often as needed
- **Allergies** - use tincture of nettle or nettle capsules as quick as possible - use allergy relief glycerite remedy
- **Anxiety** - Stress Relief Glycerite, skullcap, passionflower, valerian root capsules, chamomile tea or capsule
- **Asthma** - Lobelia tincture or mullein oil
- **Bites** - Plantain poultice, itch relief stick, or if infection or poisonous use charcoal paste or black salve
- **Boils** - Apply black salve or plantain poultice
- **Broken Bones** - Comfrey poultice and / or comfrey tea
- **Bronchial** - Mullein Oil or inhaling the smoke of mullein leaves, steam inhalation of eucalyptus oil, rosemary oil, or peppermint oil
- **Burns** - Calendula salve or Miracle salve, lavender oil
- **Cold** - Immune Boost Formula, elderberry tincture or glycerite or cold capsules
- **Congestion** - Slippery Elm Ginger Lozenges, Vapour Rub, eucalyptus oil, rosemary oil, vapor shower disks
- **Cough** - Slippery Elm Ginger Lozenges, Elderberry syrup, echinacea and Goldenseal capsules
- **Dehydration** - Rehydration formula
- **Deep Wounds** - Neosporin ointment, plantain poultice, miracle salve, calendula salve, geranium oil for clotting
- **Ear aches** - Mullein oil, garlic oil, oregano oil, or St. John's wort oil in ears, and echinacea and goldenseal capsules
- **Ear infections** - Same as ear aches
- **Eczema** - Milk thistle seed tincture for liver detox, Balm of Gilead or calendula salve topical
- **Fever** - Yarrow tea or yarrow capsules
- **Flu**- Immune boost formula, echinacea and goldenseal tincture or capsules, yarrow tea or

capsules for fever

- **Headaches** - Migraine tincture, lobelia tincture or capsules, arnica salve applied topically, valerian root capsules, lavender oil, arnica oil,

- **Heartburn** - marshmallow tea or capsule, mullein tea or capsule, peppermint tea after eating

- **Heart attack** - cayenne pepper capsule, powder or tincture

- **Infections** - internally goldenseal, echinacea, usnea, for bladder or urinary - uva ursi, topically plantain poultice, miracle salve, neosporin or black salve, tea tree oil, lavender oil, clove oil for tooth infections and aches

- **Insomnia** - valerian root capsule or tincture, chamomile tea or capsule, St. John's wort capsules, hops tincture or tea, lavender oil

- **Indigestion** - peppermint, fennel, lemon balm, lavender, all taken in capsule, tea or tincture, peppermint oil

- **Irritable Bowel** - IBS tea, or make into capsule, peppermint oil

- **Menopause** - Hot flash tea, mood swing capsules, ache capsules,

- **Menstrual Problems** - female balancing formula, black cohosh capsules, wild yam capsules, cramp bark tea, red raspberry leaf tea, evening primrose oil

- **Motion sickness** - ginger tea, tincture or capsules

- **Muscle aches** - Deep Heat Muscle Rub, Sprain muscle rub, sprain compress, arnica oil, helichrysum oil for fibromyalgia and arthritis

- **Muscle pain** - Arnica Salve, Deep Heat Muscle Rub

- **Muscle spasms** - Sprain Muscle Rub or Arnica Salve

- **Nausea** - Ginger tea, tincture or capsule, or peppermint tea, or lemon balm tea

- **Poisoning** - Activated charcoal capsules

- **Rash** - Calendula salve, Balm of Gilead, Miracle Salve

- **Restless Leg Syndrome** - Magnesium, Restless Leg Syndrome Salve, valerian root capsules internally

- **Scrapes and Cuts** - plantain poultice, calendula salve, miracle balm, neosporin

- **Sinus Infection** - sage, goldenseal, yarrow tea or capsule, and either of these as oil rubbed in, echinacea capsules internally

- **Skin problems** - Balm of Gilead, Calendula salve, Miracle Salve, nettle capsules for internal tonic long term

- **Slivers** - activated charcoal paste, or black salve, then goldenseal myrrh salve
- **Stings** - activated charcoal paste or black salve, or plantain poultice, then goldenseal myrrh salve
- **Stress** - Stress Relief Tincture or glycerite, valerian tincture or capsules, skullcap capsules, ashwaghanda capsules
- **Sunburn** - calendula salve, miracle balm
- **Wounds - Deep** - plantain poultice, not comfrey, goldenseal myrrh salve

Herbal Preparations

There are several basic ways that herbs can be prepared for use, and they can all easily be prepared right in your own home with a few basic ingredients.

These include:

• salves, creams and balms

• teas

• tinctures and glycerites

• syrups

• capsules

• compresses and poultices

Salves, Creams and Balms

One of my all time favorite healing salves is a good calendula salve. A good salve can heal a number of things and calendula salve is definitely one of these.

Salves are easy to make and easy to store. They really only require a couple of basic ingredients, an oil (usually olive) that has been infused with herbs, and some beeswax for a hardening agent. To infuse oil with some herbs is really a simple task. You can use your favorite type of oil such as olive oil, grape seed oil, almond oil, coconut oil, apricot, avocado, or other. You can even combine them if you choose. Just make sure it is a good quality oil, which will make your salve last longer and have stronger healing properties.

There are a couple of ways you can infuse the oil. Cold infusion is when you place the herbs in a glass jar and cover with oil of your choice. Stir and shake well, and allow it to sit in a warm sunny spot for four to six weeks. Shake it every day to keep it well mixed up. When time is up strain and squeeze the herbs well, and place the fresh infused oil in a clean jar for use. This is a long slow process, but if you are not in a hurry, it is a great way to create an herbal infused oil and soak as much of the healing properties from the herbs.

Hot oil infusion is a much quicker way get the end product. You prepare the herbs and oil just the same as you would with the cold infusion, but place your glass jar in a pot of water on the stove, or in a crock pot that has a couple of inches of water in the bottom, on lowest setting. You don't want to bring the oil to a boil, but let it steep on low heat for several hours or up to 3 days. Make sure you add water as it evaporates. If you are worried that the jar might break, you can place a small towel on the bottom of the pot in the water. I have also placed the herbs and oil straight into the top of a double boiler and let them heat on low for an hour or two. This is the quickest method if you are in a hurry, but again be careful not to let the oil come to a boil. The herbs will be crispy when you go to strain them out, but that is what they are supposed to be like. There really is no right or wrong way to do it as far as hot or cold infusion. Both work well.

When you are finished with your herbal infused oil, you are then ready to create your salve. Make sure your oil is strained well, and then place back into a pot on low heat. Add your grated beeswax. A good rule of thumb to follow is ½ cup of grated beeswax per cup of oil. I tend to add a bit more beeswax rather than too little because I have found that during the summer heat, these salves will melt all over the place if you don't have enough beeswax in the end product. To know if you have enough wax in your product you can test a sample quickly by taking a teaspoon full of your melted salve and stick it in the freezer for a few minutes. It will set quickly and you will be able to feel of the consistency to see if you need to add more.

Lip Balms, and deodorants are created basically the same way as the salves. Some of these will add essential oils and other types of oils or butters. Just follow the recipes that you find, or some of them listed here and they are really surprisingly easy to create, remembering if you live in a hot area, you will want to add a bit more beeswax. I have a few of these listed in the remedies section, for itching, bites, bugs, and such.

Teas

I am sure that the art of tea making goes back to the beginning of time. It is one of the easiest and best ways to get the medicinal properties of herbs into your system in a quick way. A good guide to follow when creating herbal teas is using 1 tablespoon of dried herbs to 1 cup of water. If the herbs are fresh you will want to double that amount. There are two ways to make teas: decoctions and infusions.

Decoctions are made by taking an herb, usually a root part that is tough, and boiling it for several minutes to an hour, to pull the properties out of the herb. This is usually used for roots, barks, seeds and tough herbs. It is not really a convenient way to use herbs for first aid because of the length of time it takes. Usually for first aid, these types of herbs will be used as tinctures because they can be already made. You can look to Chapter Nine, Whole Herb Tinctures, for more information on tinctures and using them.

Infusions are like your basic tea. You simply need to pour boiling water over the herbs and let them steep for a few minutes. These can be prepared in larger quantities also and then stored in the fridge to drink cold over a period of a day or two. This is great if you are fighting an illness and you make up a big batch so that you don't have to keep boiling water each time you want to drink a cup of infusion.

Good teas to keep in your kit would include:
- Chamomile
- Feverfew
- Ginger
- Peppermint
- Echinacea
- Lavender
- Rosemary
- Fennel
- Lemon Balm

Tinctures, Glycerites, Vinegars

These are really easy to prepare, but take time to process. Tinctures are usually prepared with some form of alcohol, like vodka, that is strong and pure. Alcohol is a great preservative, and also pulls out the medicinal properties of the herbs.

Glycerites are made using 100% vegetable glycerin instead of alcohol. This is great for those who are alcohol intolerant, or children. I personally am not a fan of alcohol, and prefer to use glycerin.

It is important to know the properties of the herb that you want to be tincturing because some of them are not soluble in glycerin, only alcohol. Sometimes apple cider vinegar can replace the alcohol.

Tincturing is simple. You place the desired herb or herbs, into a glass jar. Make sure they are chopped up small. Cover with the alcohol or glycerin and let sit and brew for several weeks. Shake daily. Strain well when done and squeeze out all the liquid from the herbs. Voila! That is all there is to it.

Depending on which menstruum you use, your tincture will have a pretty long shelf life if kept out of the sun and heat. Alcohol has a longer shelf life than glycerin. An alcohol tincture will have a shelf life of up to five years, where as a glycerite will have about half of that shelf life. Again, make sure you label your tinctures well so you can keep track of the dates.

Glycerites are often called syrups because the glycerin is so sweet. They are made the same way as tinctures, but using 100% vegetable glycerin. Most often the glycerin will be mixed with a ratio of water. I like to mix mine with 75% glycerin and 25% water. I will mix the two together and then pour over the herbs waiting in the jar. Then at this point, the process is the same as described above.

Syrups are made other ways. If you make a strong tea out of the herbs you want to use, and then add sugar, and allow to boil until it thickens a bit, that is all there is to making a syrup. The normal amount of sugar or honey to add is one cup per 2 cups of liquid. Heat it all so it is dissolved and mixed well together.

Remember doing this, you don't want to bring honey to a boil because it will destroy any of its healing properties. If you use honey, you will just melt it in and stir well, and the syrup will be done. Once done, pour it into a bottle, label it well and refrigerate it. Use as needed.

Vinegars are made the same way. Apple cider vinegar will be the only vinegar you will use for making herbal medicines. It has on its own some amazing healing properties. However, the taste is not always appealing to everyone, so often the other methods are preferred.

Capsules

I love making my own herbal capsules. The first time I did this I was amazed at how little herb goes into each capsule. To purchase herbs bulk, and then capsule them yourself, saves a whole lot of money. Purchasing herbs in bulk, especially the ones that you use often, is just smart. I have a local health food store that sells some in bulk, but I also often purchase them bulk from Mountain Rose Herbs. Their prices are very inexpensive, comparatively, and they get the product to you very quick.

The most expensive part of it all is purchasing the capsules themselves. Gel caps come in different sizes, so it will make a difference if you have problems swallowing larger capsules, then you will want the small "O" size. If you want to get more herb into you, then purchase the "OO" size. Gel caps come in vegetarian gel caps, and non vegetarian. The vegetarian gel caps are slightly more expensive than the others, but then you are ensuring that you are swallowing natural vegetable ingredients. It is a personal preference, with no right or wrong type of capsule to purchase.

You will also need to purchase a capsule machine. It is a slick little machine that makes filling capsules a breeze. My kids love to fill our own capsules using this little machine. Again, your local health food store may carry these, but if they don't you can find them at The Bulk Herb Store online, along with the gel caps. It is a small investment, but once you realize how much money you will be saving by filling your own capsules, you will be glad you bought it. Making your own capsules will guarantee that you know what is going into your capsules, and how fresh the herbs are. If you can grow your own herbs, even better because then you know exactly how fresh they are, and you don't have to buy them!

Compresses and Poultices

Compresses and poultices are excellent to use in first aid situations. They get the herbs to the are quickly and effectively.

Compresses can be used on sprains, chest congestion, inflamed areas, sunburns and muscle aches. You simply soak a soft cloth in an herbal infusion and apply with some pressure to the area affected. Re-soak the cloth every ½ hour or so and reapply as needed throughout the day and night. They feel great, and work directly where needed.

Poultices are similar to compresses, but use a mash of herbs instead of an infusion. The herb is mashed fresh, or dried herb mixed with hot water. Mash it until a fine mush is made, and then apply to the injury. Cover it with some gauze or sterile bandage and wrap to keep it in place. Replace it every couple of hours as needed. Plantain poultices are one of my favorite healing poultices. They are amazing, and often free as plantain grows pretty much everywhere.

Stomach, Dehydration, Motion Sickness

Digestive problems are a common ailment with first aid. Too many people are not healthy eaters, are overweight, and have reaped the consequences of having stomach problems. Most of these stomach upsets can be treated successfully with herbal remedies. Diarrhea, constipation, indigestion, irritable bowel, and nausea, all can usually be prevented with proper health and nutrition, and all can be treated with a good herbal first aid kit. I say they can be treated with an herbal first aid kit, but that will be a short term treatment. All of these ailments stem from a more serious problem, usually due to the foods we have eaten. This can be caused by an allergic reaction to something, to how our body is processing the foods we are eating. Perhaps our bodies are not absorbing the nutrients they need from the food we are eating, or we are not feeding our bodies the nutrients they need. Regardless of the reason, the herbal first aid kit, is a quick fix to an ailment, but not a long term solution.

If you are having digestion problems, you need to do some digging and find out why. More often than not, to alleviate your digestion problems, it will take some lifestyle changes to help completely eliminate them. For the purposes of this book, we will only focus on some temporary reliefs.

A great book to purchase, that is really detailed about the digestive system and all body systems, is called "The Authentic Herbal Healer" by Holly Bellebuono. This book is great to help understand how each system of the body works and how to heal them if they are not working properly. I highly recommend having this book in your library. You will reference it often I am sure.

Indigestion

For indigestion, pretty much any of the carminative herbs will work. Carminatives will dispel the gas in the intestines. These include **lavender, mint, rosemary, juniper, ginger, licorice root, fennel, or cinnamon**. Any of these can be taken as a tea or as a tincture and will produce similar results. It depends on what your preference for tastes are, and whether you are an adult or child, as some of them will be stronger in flavor or spice, and others much more mild.

Rosemary is one of those wonderful herbs that does double duty, as it increases your digestive juices and dispels gases. Most herbs will have multiple actions that they perform, and if you understand this, you can simplify the first aid process often by using one herb to do many things, instead of having to use complicated remedies.

Include **rosemary and fennel** in your cooking and it will actually help to digest fats. Fennel and chamomile are a great combination for young children to take. It would also be important to take a tonic tincture like **Nettle** tincture 2 or 3 times per day to help heal your internal digestive system. Taking nettle capsules will provide the same results and drinking nettle tea daily is very healing. Nettle is a general healthy tonic herb that heals overall. It helps the elimination system of the body work properly. Other healthy tonics that you could consider taking regularly to help heal the digestive system would include: **lemon balm, burdock root, motherwort, and chamomile**. Tonics are herbs that can be taken long term as an overall nutritive and healing approach for either a specific system in the body or the body as a whole.

Cayenne, peppermint, fennel, lemon balm, and ginger are all great herbs to take as capsule or tincture or drink as tea to help relieve indigestion.

Chamomile is not only calming to the nervous system but it will also help calm the stomach if you drink a cup of chamomile tea. These herbs will all help to relieve gas and that bloating feeling. If you get indigestion a fair bit, then sample each herb and it's various forms of taking it and see which seems to work best for you, as well as which you like the taste of best.

Peppermint Oil diluted in a carrier oil and then rubbed on the abdomen will help to relieve Indigestion or IBS, and the cramping that goes along with these.

Herbs that help to stimulate the digestive system are called **bitters,** and **include: angelica, black cohosh, dandelion, skullcap, cayenne, lemon balm, and yarrow.** **Dandelion** is probably the most popular herb that is used as a bitter and is available already as a tea, and it grows in great abundance most places.

If you have excess stomach acid, don't use the bitter herbs, but look to the demulcent herbs such as the **marshmallow or mullein, and oats**.

Ginger, is also a good digestive aid and is number one when it comes to getting rid of nausea.

Irritable Bowel

Stress and diet are the two major contributing factors for Irritable Bowel Syndrome. If we can figure out how to reduce or even eliminate our stress, and then work hard toward eating a healthy diet, it will go a long way to eliminating this common ailment that so many people have. That is the long term goal. In the mean time how to do you help someone who is suffering from the symptoms of IBS?

Some of the best antispasmodic herbs for this would include: **black cohosh, chamomile, lavender, lemon balm, mint, skullcap, valerian, wild yam, and yarrow.** These all will help to nourish the digestive system. Antispasmodic's do just what the name says, they will help stop the bowel from having is spasms. They also help the stomach from cramping up. Drinking them as a tea or taking a tincture is the best way to absorb them into your system the quickest. However, capsules will work as well, just not as quickly.

IBS Tea
2 parts stinging nettle or yarrow

2 parts oatstraw

2 parts lemon balm or chamomile

1 part peppermint

This tea will help to ease the indigestion, gas and bloating feeling. Drinking this tea after eating will help to ease the IBS before it begins. Any of the antispasmodic herbs could be added into this tea and be helpful as well

Slippery Elm is a great herb to help ease diarrhea. It coats the lining to the intestinal system and adds bulk to the stool. It will also help to soften the stool, and help with constipation.

Acid Reflux, Heartburn

Demulcent herbs are herbs that will help soothe a stomach that is having acidic problems. They are known to soothe, coat and lubricate the stomach. The best herbs for this would include **marshmallow, mullein, and oats**. These can be taken as a tea, capsule, or even eaten as traditional oatmeal. Tea would be the best way to get the soothing into your system as quick as possible.

If you concern is ongoing, then perhaps you need to look at changing your eating habits. There are reasons that heartburn and acid reflux are a problem, and if you have them often, then a change of eating may be required.

Peppermint tea will help with relieving heartburn after eating. Peppermint oil or tincture will help with this as well. **Ginger tea** or tincture can help to neutralize excess acid as well. A nice cup of tea is always relaxing to both the mind and body after a long day and a heavy meal. It will help not only to neutralize excess acid, but encourage better digestion.

Nausea, Motion Sickness

Ginger Tincture, Ginger Tea, or Ginger Capsules are the number one remedy for nausea. However if ginger is not one of your favorite flavors, then peppermint tea is a great second. Rubbing **peppermint oil**, mixed in a carrier oil, on your abdomen will also help to alleviate nausea. Often just the smell of either ginger or peppermint will be sufficient to ease an upset stomach. If you are not a fan of teas or tinctures, capsules will do the trick. Take one or two capsules of either ginger or mint - usually peppermint or spearmint - and it should ease your stomach quickly.

Dehydration

Drink as much as possible when you have the flu symptoms because you don't want to get dehydrated. Dehydration can kill quickly, especially little children.

There are many recipes available for an electrolyte replacement drink, but the point of this one is that it can be packed into an herbal first aid kit for use at a later time. I would make up a batch and then put about 2 tablespoons of the mix into a small ziploc. This is enough to add to a cup of cold water and make one glass of electrolyte drink.

Rehydration Formula

2 quarts of water

1 teaspoon of baking soda

1 - 2 teaspoons of salt

6 - 8 tablespoon of sugar or honey

1 package of kool-aid

Mix it all well in a pitcher. Cool and serve. Keep drinking until your dehydration symptoms have subsided. If you use sugar instead of honey, you can even have packages made up of this in Ziploc baggies and carry them in your first aid kit, so all you need to do is add them to a bottle of water, or a glass of water and shake well.

Often dehydration is directly related to diarrhea. If this is one of the symptoms you are experiencing, there are a few herbs that can be taken to help alleviate it.

These are mild astringent herbs and include: **chamomile, raspberry leaf, plantain leaves, spearmint, and fennel seed.** If you have a tea made from one or more of these herbs, it should be sufficient to stabilize your diarrhea enough to allow the fluids to remain in your system well enough to stave off dehydration. If you feel you need a stronger astringent to do the job then the following herbs should be considered: yarrow, or blackberry bark or root. Yarrow is my personal favorite in tea form. It is very effective and powerful and can be found growing many places in the wild. Drink as much of these teas as you can to get fluids into your system to relieve the diarrhea and to avoid dehydration. Yarrow is also a great herb to fight infection and to fight fevers. It is a good choice for several symptoms that often occur with the same illness.

Bugs, Rashes, Stings, Slivers, Boils, Blisters

Our skin is kind of a tell all. It offers us many signs that something might be wrong within our body. We can feel for heat, sweating, swelling, moistness or dryness. We can see redness, rashes, swelling, scratches, wounds, eczema, infections, and other things that are indicators that we can treat.

There are many remedies that can treat the skin or symptom both externally and internally, depending on what the underlying cause might be. This chapter will cover many of these that can be treated in a first aid situation. If something you are treating is in need of further investigation, please don't hesitate to consult with your physician, or your naturopathic doctor.

Bugs, Stings, Bites

Let's face it, we all hate the little critters that like to bite us. But they are more of an irritant than a medical concern. However, in saying that, there are those that can cause us great concern, like the Brown Recluse Spider. So always find the source of your bug bites, and if it is more than one that is just an irritant like a mosquito bite or a bee sting, then you should seek medical attention right away. If you are unsure of what bit you, treat as best you can, then seek medical attention. Never leave it unattended. Too many little critters can cause big problems.

Bug repellant spray

1 ounce rubbing alcohol or witch hazel

1 ounce grape seed oil or olive oil - if infused with yarrow it will be much more effective. Add yarrow to oil and heat on low for 2 hours, or let it sit in a jar and steep for two weeks

30 drops citronella essential oil

20 drops eucalyptus essential oil, this could be substituted with tea tree oil

15 drops lemon or lemongrass or a combination essential oil

15 drops cedar essential oils

10 drops of sweet basil

10 drops of camphor - optional

Mix well in a spray bottle and use when outdoors. Spray again every couple of hours as needed. This could also be turned into a bug repellant salve. Eliminate the alcohol or witch hazel and instead use olive oil and add 1/2 again as much grated beeswax. Melt the beeswax in the olive oil, remove from heat, add essential oils, stir well, and pour into containers. Label well. Apply often as needed while outside. This is very safe for little children as well as adults.

Plantain Bite and Sting Poultice

I love plantain. It is as common almost as dandelion once you know what you are looking for. Pick some fresh plantain leaves and mash well making a poultice. You could also chew them well and apply directly to wound for immediate relief of bite or sting. It is also great for small cuts, rashes, bruises, and almost anything minor if you are outside not close to anything else. Plantain is one of the herbs that could be labelled a heal all herb.

Itch relief stick

1 ounce of olive oil (more if needed to cover herbs completely) infused with calendula flowers, chickweed, nettle leaf, lemon balm leaf, plantain leaf, and yarrow, about 2 tbsp of each

1 ounce Shea butter 2 tbsp or coconut oil will work also

1 ounce or more of beeswax 2 - 4 tbsp

2 tsp essential oil blend of citronella oil, lavender oil, rosemary oil, tea tree oil, sandalwood, chamomile

Melt all the oils, except essential oils, and butters together over low heat. Add grated beeswax and melt. Remove from heat and stir in essential oils. Stir in well and pour into a empty push up container. Use as needed for bites and rashes.

Fungal Infections, or Ringworm

Tea Tree oil is one of the most effective remedies to use as an antifungal or antiparisitical. Tea Tree oil shouldn't be used full strength so dilute it 10% Tea Tree mixed with 90% carrier oil such as olive oil or jojoba oil. Rub it over the affected area several times per day. Garlic oil is also a great antibacterial and antiviral and would work great for this along with Tea Tree, alternate treatments.

Rashes and Skin Conditions

This Calendula salve is one of the best salves going for rashes or skin irritations, including baby diaper rash. Another that rivals it is the Balm of Gilead Salve. I have included both remedies here, make them and use them, so that you can include them in your herbal first aid kit. They are both excellent.

Balm of Gilead salve is exceptionally good for eczema and dry skin conditions. The Calendula Salve is often made with just the herb calendula, but this recipe here is a great heal all, thus the name it is sometimes given, Miracle Balm. Keep in mind that eczema is a symptom of a bigger problem. Our skin is a main route to relieve our bodies of toxins, and eczema is often a sign that the liver or kidneys are not removing the toxins in our system like they should. Liver tonics and kidney tonics should be used to help for this, as well as treating the eczema topical. Liver tonics would include, milk thistle seed, burdock root, dandelion root, and nettles.

Calendula Salve or Miracle Balm

1 ¼ c olive oil or more as needed to completely cover the herbs

1/3 ounce of dried calendula flowers

1/3 ounce dried plantain

¼ ounce dried St. John's Wort

1/4 ounce dried Comfrey

¼ ounce dried Oregon grape root

1 - 2 ounces beeswax - I tend to add the greater amount so the salve doesn't melt in hot weather

Essential oils to add might be lemon, eucalyptus, lemongrass, and lavender. These all have some great healing properties, as well as great preservative properties for the salve to last longer. Infuse the herbs into the oil using the hot oil method mentioned earlier. When done strain the herbs out well. Return the oil to the pot and add the beeswax. Melt over low heat. Remove from heat and add any essential oils you might want to add. Remember with essential oils, a little goes a long way. When stirred in, pour into clean sterile containers. Allow to harden. Place on lid and label well so you know what it is or so someone else using your first aid kit will also know what to do with it.

Balm of Gilead Salve

You need to find a nice grove of poplar trees, because the "Balm of Gilead" is the resin on the buds of the poplar tree. Any type of poplar tree will do, it doesn't have to be a specific variety. Very first thing in the spring as the tree is starting to bud out, you will notice that the buds have a very sticky resin that oozes from them. This is the prime time to pick the buds. A cool day would be best because the buds aren't quite as sticky, but any time will do. Harvest yourself a cup or two of the nice swollen resinous buds. Pick a few off each branch, so you don't stress out any one particular branch of the tree. Once you have a nice stash, add them to a jar and cover them with olive oil with a couple of inches to spare, because they will swell a bit more in the oil. Let them sit in the oil for a couple of weeks up to 2 months to let the oil absorb as much of the resin as possible. Shake it well everyday because the resin will settle to the bottom of the jar.

When it is done soaking, strain it out well and gently heat the oil over a low burner. Add about 1/4 cup of grated beeswax to each cup of oil that you end up with. When it is all melted, pour into clean sterile containers and allow to harden.

** You could add some carrot seed oil to this salve - it is great for psoriasis and eczema and most skin problems. Balm of Gilead salve is also great for muscle aches and joint pains. It tends to drive deep into muscles, so can be used for any deep tissue salve.

Lavender Oil is great for skin care and healing. Diluted in a carrier oil, it can be rubbed onto rashes, burns, bruises, scrapes, acne, bug bites, and generally any skin ailment. It is gentle and soothing to the skin.

Tea Tree Oil is a great oil to have on hand for many skin conditions. When diluted with a carrier oil it is good to treat athlete's foot, acne, skin wounds, and insect bites.

Slivers, Boils, Stings, Infections, Poisoning

Activated Charcoal

Activated charcoal is great if you don't have the Black Salve available. Simply make a paste out of the charcoal and some water and paste it onto the sting, sliver, or infection and wrap it well with clean gauze or cloth. Replace often, every couple of hours, until you get the desired results.

Activated charcoal is used to treat poisoning, and help with intestinal gas, lower cholesterol, and even help prevent hangovers. It does this because it is the best at capturing chemicals and prevents their absorption into your system. Get capsules into your system as quickly as possible for poisoning. For other problems, use as needed to help you feel better, but follow the directions on the bottle if you have purchased capsules. It would be important to use capsules for these purposes, so either purchase some capsules, or make your own capsules and have them available for anytime use. Always carry activated charcoal with you in your herbal first aid kit.

Drawing Salve - Black salve

Can be applied to boils, stings, bites, slivers, and anything or anywhere that needs to draw out infection or an object. These measurements are weighted measurements, not amounts. Use your kitchen scale to weigh them.

6 ounces of olive oil infused with goldenseal, chickweed, and plantain equal parts of each

2 ounces castor oil - it has great drawing properties

1 ounce beeswax grated

½ cup activated charcoal

½ c bentonite clay

1 tsp of each essential oil, clove, rosemary, lemon, lavender, and eucalyptus

Infuse oil over the stove with the herbs for a couple of hours. Strain well and return to stove on low heat. Stir in beeswax until melted. Remove from heat and stir in castor oil, charcoal, clay, and essential oils. Stir and mix well. Pour into a glass jar or tins and label well. Store in a cool dark place. Place small amount of salve to affected area and keep bandaged for 12 hours, redoing every 2 hours until healed. This stuff is amazing.

Goldenseal Myrrh salve

- for after use of black salve to help aid in preventing infection and promote healing.

1 part Goldenseal Root

1 part Comfrey Root

1 part Calendula Petals

1 part Echinacea Root

1 part Myrrh Resin - Powdered

Virgin Olive Oil - enough to cover the herbs and a bit plus. Infuse in oil for 3 – 4 weeks or use quick method.

Beeswax - about 1/2 as much grated beeswax as olive oil, or a little bit less

Vitamin E - about 1 tsp per quart of oil. To be added after melting beeswax and removed from heat. It is a great preservative and healing agent.

Complete Tissue Repair Ointment by Dr. Kyle Christensen in his book Herbal First Aid and Health Care. This is such a great recipe to heal almost anything. Use on any external injury and watch miracles take place. Infuse the herbs into a pure olive oil. Then create a salve using pure beeswax.

6 parts comfrey root, and white oak bark

3 parts each: marshmallow root, mullein, black walnut bark, gravel root

2 parts each: wormwood, white willow bark

1 part each: St. John's wort, lobelia, skullcap, horsetail

Calendula Salve is another salve that is a heal all. It is great for burns, infections, rashes, bites, small scrapes and wounds. It is just a great healing salve.

<u>Kloss's Herbal Liniment</u> a great ointment very popular and recipe readily available in most herb books and web sites.

1 ounce echinacea powder

1 ounce goldenseal root powder

2 ounces myrrh gum powder

½ ounce cayenne pepper powder

rubbing alcohol to cover - approximately 1 quart

Place herbs in a clean glass jar. Fill with rubbing alcohol leaving an inch head space. Mix and blend well. Let stand in a warm spot for about 4 weeks. This is different from a tincture because it is only to be used externally. Make sure it is clearly labelled this way. After it has steeped for 4 weeks, strain well and bottle. Label well. This liniment can be applied every few minutes for an hour or two in acute instances. Use freely until desired results. If bottled in spray bottles it is really easy to use. This liniment is so powerful it will stop a stye from developing on the eye by dabbing on with a q tip. Don't get in eye. By applying to temples, back of neck, and to forehead it can e used as an excellent remedy for a headache. Spray on swollen joints or arthritis spots for relief. Can also be used on cuts, ringworm, sprains, sunburn, poison ivy, and chicken pox.

Infections

There are are a few antibacterial herbs that are great to help treat infections and can be added to any salves or taken internally as tinctures or capsules.

Antibacterial herbs include: **goldenseal, oregon grape root, Echinacea, elecampane, usnea, and marshmallow.**

The Calendula salve, Black salve, and the Neosporin salve are all good ones to use for exterior infections.

Tooth infections - use **clove oil**

Tea Tree Oil - has been used and effective treating against Staphylococcus and fungal infections. It is highly antibacterial, antiviral, and anti fungal.

Internal infections **- basil and oregano** are some of the most healing herbs that you can take internally to heal fungus or infections within.

Basil oil is highly inhibitory at restricting the growth of bacteria strains, including Staph and E-coli infections. You could add some drops of oil to water and drink it to help heal internally, and for externally, add drops of the oil to a carrier oil like almond or olive and rub into the area where it is needed.

Oregano oil has extreme anti-fungal, anti-bacterial, and anti-viral properties. It is proven to to kill most infections both internal and external. It is really a strong potent oil, so always dilute it before you rub it on your skin or it could burn you. Also dilute it in a small amount of water before drinking it. It is also available in gel caps in most health food stores, so this also is an option and a good thing to have on hand because the taste of this oil is very strong.

Kidney or urinary tract infections

Drink as many cups of this tea per day as you can. The more the better. Try to drink a full gallon of tea each day. This formula can be drank as tea or made into a tincture.

2 parts juniper berries

1 part each: uva ursi leaf, usnea, dandelion leaf, orange peel, peppermint, gravel root, marshmallow root. Use 1 tsp of dried herb per cup of boiling water. Drink lots to heal and flush the bladder and kidneys.

Cranberry juice is also a great drink because it helps make the walls of the bladder slippery so the bacteria can't attach itself and it just gets flushed out.

Blisters

Saturate a small piece of gauze with witch hazel. Place it over the blister with some medical tape. When the blister opens, clean it with Kloss's liniment and an equal part of water. Apply comfrey / calendula salve and cover with a bandage. This will heal the blister quickly.

Cuts, Wounds, Scrapes, Burns, Rashes

Our skin is the largest organ of our body, and tell tale that something is wrong with our body. It will give us indicators, like heat, swelling, rashes, and sweat.

Often when dealing with first aid situations, we will treat something that has to do with the skin. It might be a cut, puncture, scrape, rash, burn, infection, eczema, muscle, bone, sting, and so forth, but we treat it through the skin.

Wounds require a different healing tactic that some other skin problems such as burns and rashes. Some herbs are great for healing surface wounds, and some are used for deeper healing. If you have a deep puncture wound, it would be wise to seek medical attention as soon as you get a chance. It really isn't fun to attempt to give yourself stitches, and you will likely cause more damage than good. Infection will often set in, in a deep puncture wound if it is not treated properly.

Our wound healing herbs are called vulneraries. This term came about from the idea that if you are vulnerable, you can be hurt, and therefore herbs that heal are called vulnerary.

Yarrow and comfrey are two herbs that are excellent at healing surface wounds. They go to work quickly and effectively to seam wounds back together. Herbs to help fight infection of a wound might include: yarrow, thyme, and goldenseal.

Healing wounds is one area that herbs seem to just excel.

Wounds and Skin Problems

Along with the many other salves and remedies that we have already discussed, that could be included in this chapter, we have a couple of more.

Previous ones that should be listed here include: calendula salve, lavender salve, plantain poultice, miracle balm, balm of gilead, black salve, and more.

Neosporin is a natural antibiotic topical ointment, similar to the one that can be purchased at the pharmacy. The oils used in it are great healers, antibiotics, antibacterial, and antifungal. It is a great ointment and can be used on any age of patient.

Neosporin ointment

3 cups olive oil

1 c grated beeswax

1/4 c comfrey leaf

1/4 c plantain leaf

1/4 c calendula petals

1/8 c yarrow

1 tsp vitamin E oil or grapefruit seed oil - acts as a preservative

1 tsp tea tree oil

20 drops lavender essential oil

10 drops lemon essential oil

Melt oil and beeswax over low heat. Remove from heat and add vitamin E oil and essential oils. Stir well. Pour into small jars or containers. Use as you would a neosporin or polysporin or antiseptic ointment.

Some different herbs to think about when making your salves. Include what you feel you need, or create a salve with a single herb. Mix and match them to create your family's own special miracle salves.

A salve made with **Goldenseal** is a great antiseptic and antibiotic and would be great for infections, minor cuts and scrapes, chapped skin or other skin irritations.

Chamomile is both anti-inflammatory and antiseptic and wonderful for itch relief.

Bloodroot is a very potent herb! Salve made with bloodroot is typically call black salve. This herb has an amazing drawing ability. This herb is not for beginners but definitely worth mentioning.

Chickweed is a great remedy for any type of itchy skin condition. Use for bug bites and stings, chicken pox, measles, rashes or simply dry skin.

Calendula is best known for its skin healing properties. Calendula is a very gentle yet effective herb to use in combination with any other salve herb.

Arnica is world renown as a pain reliever. Try some arnica salve on your temples for headaches, and remember never take internally

Lemon balm salve is excellent for anyone who gets frequent cold sores, and can be added into any salve for great aroma and relaxing properties.

Burns

Burns vary in degree, from a mild sunburn (a fourth degree burn) to a 1st degree burn which burns right through and affects deep muscle tissue and possible bones. Every degree of burn is dangerous and should be treated carefully. If you have received a serious burn, medical attention should be sought immediately. Mild burns are all we really can deal with in our own home first aid.

We can treat burns after medical attention has been received, but for the purpose of this book, we will deal with the sunburns, or small burns that should and can be treated safely at home.

There are a few really great herbs that treat burns so well. Three are at the top of the list. Aloe Vera gel, Calendula salve, and Lavender oil or salve. These can be used as often as needed to heal the burn. Calendula salve is number one in my books to heal general sunburns. It shows amazing results all the time. Some love the smell of lavender as it has a relaxing, soothing smell, and its healing burn properties are also quite amazing. And we are all familiar with the Aloe Vera plant. Gel from this plant can be purchased and kept in your first aid kit, or you can try your hand at raising the plant as a house plant. It is a very forgiving plant and seems to thrive on neglect. Any or all of these should be a part of your herbal first aid kit.

Lavender Salve

1 cup lavender buds

2 cups grape seed oil

1 cup grated beeswax

30 drops lavender essential oil

Infuse the dried lavender buds in the grape seed oil. Olive oil could also be used. When done, strain the oil well and place it in a pot on the low burner setting. Add the grated beeswax. When it is melted, remove from heat and allow to cool slightly. Add the lavender oil and mix well. Pour into containers and label well.

Calendula Salve

3 cups olive oil

1 cup calendula petals

1/2 cup comfrey

1/2 cup St. John's wort

1 cup grated beeswax - or more if harder salve is desired lavender essential oil - 20 drops - optional

Infuse the herbs into the oil. Make salve with the oil. This is a great healing salve for small cuts, bruises and is simply amazing for healing sunburns. It is not good for deep cuts because of the comfrey. Comfrey will heal the outside of the wound too quickly and often the deep tissue isn't healed so infection can occur.

Muscles, Broken Bones

Muscles and bones are parts of our body that can be treated easily with natural first aid. They are often the concern for first aid due the fact that they are a major portion of our body. Remember always to seek medical attention if a joint is extremely swollen or seems out of alignment, or if you think something is broken.

Arnica is a great healing and pain relieving herb. It has shown to reduce healing time by half. Don't use it on an open wound though, as it can cause irritation to the mucus membranes.

With broken bones, nettles will provide essential healing minerals for bone regeneration. Take the capsules daily or drink the tea daily. Two other herbs that will do this as well are: oatstraw and horsetail. These are long term herbs to take to help provide the healing process and your body, the vital minerals it needs.

Muscles

Deep Heat Muscle Rub

Make a salve using the following herbs infused into olive oil and hardened with beeswax.

1 cup St. John's wort

1 cup skullcap

2 tbsp cayenne pepper

3 cups olive oil

1 cup grated beeswax - or more if you want a firmer salve

30 or 40 drops of wintergreen essential oil

This can also be used as an oil rub, just eliminate the beeswax and use it as a massage oil. But when using as an oil, be careful it will stay on your hands and the cayenne can burn when rubbed into eyes or nose or face.

Sprain Compress

A compress of St. John's Wort, witch hazel, skullcap, valerian, arnica, and chamomile will help a sprain to feel better and heal rapidly. This combination could also be made into an infused oil rub especially for sprained or strained muscles. If you make it into an oil rub, then you could carry it in your herbal first aid kit and label it Sprained Muscle Rub. Then rub it into muscle sprain as often as needed and wrap with a bandage to keep the oils against the muscle and away from your clothing.

Sprain Muscle Rub

Equal parts: St. John's wort, skullcap, valerian, arnica, chamomile

Infuse in Olive oil then strain well when complete. Label well, and label that it is only for external use. Arnica is not to be used internally.

Back Spasm or Pain

Use the Sprain Muscle Rub for back spasms or pain. The chamomile and skullcap are great for easing inflammation and helping to heal the sore muscle, and the St. John's wort is great for calming the anxiety and stress surrounding the muscles and in you.

Peppermint Oil diluted in a carrier oil and then massaged into aching muscles and painful joints can help relieve the affected area.

A **Lobelia tincture** could also be used as a muscle relaxant. It can also be used in a pill form that you can get from the health food store, or again make your own capsules. It is often used to ease muscle cramps and spasms. It has also been used to treat migraines effectively. Lobelia does have a caution though, and should not be used too much. Overuse can cause vomiting, so use in moderation and only when needed.

Arnica oil - arnica is an herb that can reduce the healing time of an injury by half, however avoid it on an open wound because it can cause irritation. Olive oil infused with dried arnica flowers. Prepare infusion and bottle and label well. This can be stored for up to a year or longer. Arnica is one of the best pain relievers for sprains and sore muscles. Apply to bruises and sore muscles for fast relief and reduce swelling. Don't use on broken skin.. Label well. Arnica is not to be taken internally.

Arnica Salve
2 cups coconut oil
.6 ounces dried arnica flowers
½ cup beeswax grated - this will make a really soft salve so add twice this if you want a firmer salve
¼ tsp. peppermint essential oil (optional)
¼ tsp. lavender essential oil (optional)

Arnica Cayenne Salve

2 cups coconut oil

.6 ounces dried arnica flowers

4 tbsp dried cayenne powder

½ cup beeswax grated - add more if you prefer a firmer salve, this will yield a soft

salve

½ tsp. rosemary essential oil (optional)

Infuse the coconut oil with the dried arnica by heating on low for overnight. Before you add the arnica to the coconut oil, you could chop it up a bit finer in your blender. This will help the infusion happen quicker. You can refer back to Chapter 1 for more on how to infuse the oil, if you need to. If you are making the cayenne salve, you can add it to the oil and arnica at this point as well. Stir them often to help the process along. Let it infuse for a good 12 - 24 hours making sure it doesn't get too hot. If the oil gets too hot, it will destroy some of the healing properties in the coconut oil. Don't let it come to a boil, just keep it warm – hot. When it is done, strain the herbs out using a cheese cloth or a strainer, squeezing well to remove all the liquid you can. Return it to your pot on low heat and add the beeswax until it is completely melted. Remove from the heat when melted. Allow to cool slightly before adding essential oils. Pour into containers and label well. Use as a topical pain reliever on aching muscles, bruises, sprains, headaches, etc.

Broken Bones

Seek medical attention as soon as possible if you suspect a broken bone. In the mean time, if you can't get medical help, splint, wrap, sling, or contain the bone that is broken so it won't get moved or bumped. A poultice of comfrey leaf or root, or both, will help the healing begin right away. Even while the bone is cast and continued healing, drink a comfrey tea 2 or 3 times per day. Comfrey is known as "bone knit" because it goes straight to work healing broken bones and the tissue around them. In Dr. Christensen's book Herbal First Aid and Health Care, he has a great deal of information on setting different bones and how to wrap them properly. It would be good to study this and know it, to save causing more damage than good.

Also to consider, in the first aid situation of a broken bone, you may want to administer a tea or capsules of herbs that will help to **calm nerves and ease the pain.** Often if there is a broken bone, there will be some sort of shock as well.

Shock can be treated with nervine herbs which would include: St. John's wort, lemon balm, chamomile, or skullcap. Any of these herbs would be great to administer in tea, tincture, or capsule form to help ease anxiety and shock.

For the pain, a good analgesic herb should be administered, in tea, tincture, or capsule form again. These might include: willow bark, chamomile, St. John's wort, chickweed, hops or passionflower. Externally you should apply one of the following Arnica salves. This is greatly know for pain relieving and reducing inflammation in muscles. Arnica should never be taken internally.

Colds, Flu, Sinus, Fever, Asthma, Allergies

Herbal medicine has a long history of treating respiratory problems. The respiratory system includes the ears, sinus, throat, lungs, and everything that has to do with them. Some herbs are great for drying up mucous, some for fevers, some for coughs, and some for pain related to them all. Perhaps the most common herb for fighting respiratory problems that we know, is Echinacea. Again, the caution is if you have any concerns about a problem, don't hesitate to seek medical advice. Herbal medicine can treat a cough and sore throat, but if it doesn't get better after a couple of treatments, be aware of Strep. Strep can become quite serious and cause damage if it doesn't get treated with an antibiotic, so never let it go unattended. Another caution is ear infections. Ear infections can easily be treated with herbal remedies, but if for some reason they don't seem to respond, seek medical attention. An ear infection, if out of control, can actually cause infection in the brain, and lead to brain damage. This would be an extreme case, however, let's not ever let it get to this point.

A good thing to remember, when treating the respiratory system, is that it is a part of the whole body. We can treat the symptoms in a first aid situation, and it will help bring relief, but the whole body system must always be considered. To completely heal from an infection, or virus, the whole body must be treated and regain it's health

Asthma, Bronchial and Ears

Ears

There are a few really great oils that can be used for an ear ache or infection, if you catch it right away. You can use a single oil, or combine the oils that you have to create an oil with the specific properties you feel you need.

Mullein oil, which is olive oil infused with mullein. A few warm drops of this oil dropped in the troubled ear, should quickly bring relief and fight off an infection. Mullein is a great antibacterial, with demulcent and astringent properties. This means that it will help fight infection, soothe the inflamed condition, and help dry up the mucous. Mullein will help to alleviate the pressure, burning and pain. Can be used on children and adults.

Garlic oil is another good one for ear infections. Again, infuse the olive oil with chopped fresh garlic for a couple of weeks on the counter, shaking daily. Strain out the garlic and bottle the oil. Label it well. Warm a few drops before dropping into an ear that hurts. Keep applying every couple hours as needed. Garlic is a strong antibacterial, antifungal, and antiviral. It is also a great expectorant. This means that it will kill pretty much any infection and whatever is causing it. As an expectorant properties, it will cause the excess fluid and infection to drain from the ear. Good for children and adults.

Oregano oil is a really strong oil and for really bad cases of infection it can be used in the ear. It really is pretty strong so be careful using this oil for children. If you do use it, never use it straight, always dilute it with a carrier oil. Then drop a couple of drops in the infected ear. Oregano is a really strong antibacterial, anti fungal, and expectorant. It will kill the bacteria causing the infection and help to expel the excess fluid and mucous from the ear.

St. John's wort is another great oil for fighting viruses and bacterias. Soak a cotton ball and place in ear, and take capsules or tinctures to fight it from the inside out. You can also massage a bit of the oil around the ear and any area of the throat that is feeling sore.

Internally for treating the ear, **Echinacea and goldenseal** tincture or capsules are great to take. They will help fight the ear infection and anywhere else the infection might be attacking. Goldenseal is a great antibacterial and anti fungal as is Echinacea. Echinacea will help to stimulate the immune system to fight the infection on its own. Take both of these herbs at the first sign of a cold, flu, or infection and keep taking it until the symptoms have gone. These are not long term herbs, so are perfect for first aid situations as they work hard and strong right away.

Sinus infection

There are a few herbs that are really great for helping with a sinus infection. Any of the herbs that are strong astringents or anticatarrhals will work to help dry up the mucous and fight the build up of mucous. Astringents will dry it up and anticatarahals are really strong astringents that work directly to dry up mucous secretions in the respiratory tract. These would include: **sage, goldenseal, yarrow, shepherd's purse, and eyebright**. Any of these herbs can be drank as a tea, taken as capsules or tinctures, and massaged into the sinus area gently.

Fight it from the inside and out by massaging, and taking the capsules. A hot compress made from one of the herbs will also be great to place over the sinus area. It will help to drain and ease the pressure. Also with a sinus infection, **Echinacea and goldenseal** will help fight the infection from the inside. Start taking at the first sign of infection and it will go straight to work.

Asthma and Bronchial

Lobelia tincture is the thing to have on hand for an acute asthma attack. 1 dropperful can stop an acute attack quickly.

Mullein oil is a strong remedy for bronchial congestion. Mullein oil will stop coughs, break up the bronchial tubes and help clear up asthma attacks.

Comfrey tea 2 - 3 times each day will also help deep healing of the lungs.

Eucalyptus Oil used as a steam inhalation can be very beneficial to congestion of the lungs, throat, and sinus. It can be used as a steam inhalation, in massage oil that can be massaged on your sinus area or chest and throat, or in the bath and shower. Below is a recipe for shower vapor disks that can be simply tossed into the bottom of the tub while showering and it will melt and give off a great steam vapor that will help with congestion.

Vapour Shower Disks

2 cups baking soda give or take depending on how much you want to make water to make a thick paste by adding a little at a time and mixing well

25 drops of eucalyptus essential oils, peppermint could also be added

Spoon these into a muffin tin lined with small muffin liners. Allow to sit out until really hard. Usually 24 hours is sufficient. Store them in a Ziploc bag in your bathroom. When you feel congested, pop them out of the liners and throw one in the bath tub or the bottom of the shower. If they have problems sticking together, you can bake them for 20 minutes at 350, but if you do this, add the essential oils to the hardened disk after baking. Heat will evaporate the essential oils as they bake.

Tea Tree Oil can be used as a steam inhalation to help relieve respiratory congestion. Keep away from eyes if you can because it can be irritating. It is very strong.

For a sore throat - Slippery Elm can be extremely soothing. It has great lubricating properties. Drink as a tea, or make some cough drops that can be sucked on when a sore throat shows up.

Slippery Elm Ginger Lozenges

1 tsp dried chopped licorice root

1/2 tsp ginger powdered

1/2 cup slippery elm powder

2 tbsp honey

Make a licorice tea by adding the root and ginger to 1/2 cup of water and boil, simmering for 10 minutes. Strain well. Using a 1/4 cup measure add the honey and fill with tea. Add this to 1/2 cup slipper elm powder and make a smooth dough. Roll this dough out to about 1/4 inch thickness. Use a cap of a bottle to cut out small circles. Place these on a tray and allow them to dry for a couple of days until they are really hard. Place in an airtight container and use as needed when a sore throat comes.

Cold and Flu

Immune Boost Formula - there are many different formulas that will boost your immunity. Use this formula to make a tincture with vodka or glycerin and water, depending on if you are alcohol intolerant or making it for children.

9 parts echinacea root

3 parts goldenseal

1 part each: siberian ginseng root, usnea, fresh garlic, peppermint

For maintenance you could use a couple of dropperfuls each day. Then at first signs of illness up this to 1 - 2 dropperfuls every hour until symptoms stop. Follow the guidelines for making tinctures and glycerites.

Elderberry syrup

1 cup of dried elderberries

3 cups water

1 cup honey

2 tbsp grated ginger root

Simmer berries and ginger in water over low heat for 45 minutes. Smash the berries well. Strain through a cheesecloth. Add honey and stir well. Bottle syrup and store in fridge for up to 3 months. Use as needed for coughs and colds. This is a great immune booster. 1 tsp per day for prevention for children. 1 tsp per hour at first signs of cold and flu. Adults 1 tbsp.

Elderberry glycerite

1 cup vegetable glycerin

1 cup water

1 1/2 cups dried berries

In a quart jar place dried elderberries. Mix the glycerin and water together and pour over berries. Shake daily for 4 - 6 weeks. The longer, the more potent. Strain well squeezing out all of the liquid. Store in an airtight container for up to six months on the shelf. **Good and safe for pregnant mothers and infants**. 1 tsp daily for prevention and 4 tsp daily at first signs of illness.

Cold and Flu Tincture or Glycerite

2 ounces dried echinacea root

1 ounce goldenseal

1 ounce yarrow

1 ounce elderberries

1 ounce dried lemon balm

1 ounce dried horehound

vodka or a mix of 60% vegetable glycerin and 40% water, enough to fill a jar. Steep in jar for 2 - 6 weeks, shaking daily. Vodka tincture will be good for 5 years on the shelf. The glycerite will be about half that shelf life.

Adults at first sign of colds ¼ - ½ tsp every 30 minutes to hour until symptoms subside. For children reduce the amount. This glycerite is safe for all ages.

Cold Capsules / super immune support

1 part Echinacea root powder

1 part rose hips powder

1 part goldenseal powder

1/2 part turmeric powder

¼ part cayenne pepper powder

Mix well and make capsules using capsule machine. At first sign of being sick take 1 - 2 capsules every 2 - 3 hours. Continue for 2 days then reduce dosage to 6 capsules a day until better.

Fever Tea

yarrow

peppermint

elder flowers

Add equal parts of each herb. Keep in a container until needed. Pour boiling water over 1 tbsp of tea mix and drink. Small children 1 - 2 tsp of tea. Adults ½ - 1 cup every 30 minutes until fever breaks. Can be made in large batches and used throughout the day as needed for easier using. It is good cold as well as hot.

Vapour Rub

1 cup of olive oil melted with 1/2 cup of beeswax

Add 2 tsp eucalyptus oil

2 tsp peppermint oil

2 tsp thyme oil

Pour into containers and let harden. Use for nasal congestion and common cold symptoms. Use for flu, coughs on chest, and sinus headaches. It is great to rub on chest, back, feet, under nose and on your temples. It does a great job of opening up the sinuses.

Allergies

Nettle capsules or tinctures are a great remedy for allergies as they contain a natural histamine. A good capsule if you can make some is a combination of nettle, astragalus, marshmallow, and ephedrine. You can make a child's allergy medicine by making a glycerite of nettles, marshmallow and astragalus, adding in some peppermint, cinnamon, or lemon balm for flavouring.

Never take chances with allergic reactions. Some reactions can be so severe they will threaten your life. Seek medical attention immediately. For mild allergies, like a hay fever reaction, nettle capsules are the best bet for allergy relief. It contains high amounts of quercetin which is used in treatment for allergies.

Allergy Glycerite
1 part nettles
1 part marshmallow
1 part astragalus
1 part lemon balm
Combine all herbs well in a glass jar and cover with 75% vegetable glycerin mixed with 25% water. Allow to sit on counter for 3 or 4 weeks shaking daily. Strain herbs well and place tincture in a clean container. Use for allergy relief.

Anxiety, Stress, Pain, Sleep, Headaches, Heart

Everyone feels overwhelmed or stressed at some point. In fact 1 in 5 teenagers suffer from serious anxiety and panic attacks. It is so easy to feel like we want to just opt out of events to avoid the anxiety caused by them. We lead these fast paced lives that have become the norm, and then we medicate to avoid the side effects, and this has become the norm.

This is a vicious cycle that is hard to break and leads to more and more symptoms and side effects, all simply from the stressful life we lead. These symptoms and side effects often include aching muscles, chronic headaches, insomnia, depression, chronic fatigue, mood swings, memory loss, high blood pressure, weight loss or gain, IBS, and decreased sexual drive. We want to treat the symptoms, and we can, but we really should be looking at the underlying cause of what the symptoms are from if we want to completely stop them.

Stress and anxiety need long term lifestyle changes. So keep in mind as we are treating the symptoms, using herbal first aid, it is only a band aid in the grand scheme of things. Figure out what the whole picture is and work towards healing that.

Anxiety, Stress and Insomnia

Stress Relief

Make a tincture or glycerite from the following.

2 parts valerian root

1 part each: passionflower, hops flowers, skullcap, wild yam. Can be used for adults or children. Good to use for tension and muscle spasm, insomnia, relaxation, anxiety and panic.

Calming Spray

2 ounces of water

20 drops of rosemary oil

20 drops of lavender oil

Combine and shake well in a spray bottle. Spray whenever calming is needed. Shelf stable, no need to refrigerate and will last indefinitely. Rosemary will help relieve headaches and tension. Lavender is proven to reduce stress and anxiety. Carry a bottle with you everywhere. You can spray it in the air and just breath or spray it onto your neck or head or wherever you feel it works best for you. It can also be sprayed directly onto your tongue for fast relief.

Chamomile tea is a great remedy to relieve a stress filled day. You could also fill some capsules and keep them handy.

Valerian Tincture

Valerian is one of stinkiest herbs I have ever smelled, but boy does it work. It has great antispasmodic properties and is a great painkiller too. It will relieve intestinal cramps, and cramps associated with women's cycles. It is great for headaches, general aches, pains, and will bring on sleep when nothing else will.

2 parts valerian root

½ part hop flowers

100 proof vodka or 60% glycerin and 40% water

Tincture for 2 - 6 weeks shaking daily. Strain well. Store in clean jar in dark place. It will keep for up to five years.

Licorice Root contains a natural hormone alternative to cortisone, which can help the body handle stressful situations, and can help to normalize blood sugar levels as well as your adrenal glands, providing you with the energy necessary to deal with the stressful situation at hand. Some claim licorice stimulates cranial and cerebro spinal fluid, thereby calming the mind. You have to be a bit careful with licorice because it will also raise your blood pressure.

Any of the nervine or anxiolytic herbs can be taken in capsule formula to help relive stress or anxiety. The more common ones include: St. John's wort (which is good for kids and pregnant mothers), skullcap, valerian root, lemon balm (also good for kids and pregnant mothers), passionflower, rosemary, lavender, and hops. Follow the directions on the labels of the bottles.

Mood Booster - for seasonal depression

1 part hawthorn
1 part oat tops
1 part lemon balm
1 part St. John's wort
Combine and mix well. Powder in blender. Make capsules and take them daily as needed.

Insomnia

Insomnia is one of the greatest problems that so many people deal with. When we don't get a good nights sleep it throws off so many other areas of our world. Chronic insomnia is suffered by approximately 1/5 of our population. Sometimes there are lifestyle changes that need to be made, and often stress is the number one cause of insomnia. So reduce the stress and hopefully sleep better. If you have problems sleeping and it is an ongoing problem, do your research to figure out what you need to change to help break the chronic cycle. In the mean time, there are some herbal medicines that help with sleeping.

Chamomile is a great mild sedative that can be taken by children and adults and is safe for pregnancy as well. It can be taken as tea, tincture, capsule, or massage oil. How about making a chamomile / hops pillow sachet to sleep on, that would help nicely.

Hops has a long history of medicine use for insomnia, anxiety, and nervousness.

Lavender Oil can be diluted and rubbed into the neck, back or temples to help relieve stress and anxiety. It will also help to relieve insomnia. It has a really pleasant and soothing smell and is gentle on skin.

Several other great ones are **valerian, passionflower, skullcap, and St. John's wort.** Try them so you know what works best and what you think of each and then you will be more ready to suggest for others. They can also be combined to work better. Often when I am feeling like I can't sleep I will take valerian and chamomile, and even throw in a St. John's wort. It always helps me relax and will bring on sleep.

Headaches

Migraine Tincture

3 parts lemon balm

3 parts feverfew

2 parts valerian root

1 part St. John's wort

100 proof vodka or 60% glycerin and 40% water to fill jar tincture for 2 -6 weeks. Strain, bottle and store for up to 5 years. At the first signs of a migraine take ½ tsp every 30 minutes to an hour until symptoms subside.

Lobelia Tincture or Capsules

Lobelia is often used as a migraine or headache relief. It can be used as a tincture or in capsule form. Follow the instructions carefully because if over used it can cause nausea and vomiting. But used in moderation it is great for relieving headaches. For more chronic headaches a person should dig to the root of the problem and treat with herbs accordingly.

Lavender Oil - is a great mild pain reliever. Just inhaling the scent is often sufficient to stave off a headache if it is caught soon enough. Dilute some with a carrier oil and then rub into the temples or the back of the neck to help relieve stress and headaches due to tension.

Peppermint Oil diluted with a carrier oil and then rubbed into the temples or massaged on the neck or area of pain can help to relieve headaches, especially caused by stress or tension.

Arnica is an herb that is widely used for topical pain relief. These recipes will help reduce inflammation and pain by rubbing salve on skin. It will help to stimulate blood flow to the area of application, which in turn will help to aid in healing.

Heart

Cayenne Tincture

A cayenne tincture could well be one of the most important items in your first aid kit if you come across someone who is having a heart attack. Kyle D. Christensen, in his book Herbal First Aid and Health Care says this "Herbally, give the person 1 to 10 dropperfuls of Cayenne tincture orally. Often the cayenne is enough to pull someone out of an acute heart attack before any permanent damage to the heart is done. Even if the person is unconscious 1 to 2 dropperfuls of cayenne can be put into the mouth. Rest causes the oxygen requirement of the heart to be at a minimum. Don't give him anything to drink. Remain calm, and try to reassure him." I highly recommend this book. Well worth keeping in your first aid kit and reading it over and over.

Cayenne Pepper

Cayenne pepper can be used to help stop any external or internal bleeding, as well as to arouse a person back to into being conscious if they tend to drift away. Tincture can be dropped under tongue, this will help with consciousness or internal bleeding. Cayenne pepper put directly on a bleeding wound will help stop the bleeding also. It may hurt a bit, but does the job.

Restless Leg

Restless leg syndrome is such a huge problem for so many people. Approximately 5% of the adult population deals with some sort of this, 2 percent of children struggle with it each night. It seems to affect women more than men, by almost twice as much. The causes are not completely know, but it has been linked to a few things like genetics, some chronic diseases, medications, pregnancy, and a possibility of lack of magnesium.

Restless Leg Syndrome Salve

1 part devils claw

1 part skullcap

1 part chamomile

1 part St. John's wort

Infuse some olive oil or your favorite other oil, with these herbs into this oil. Once they have been infused, strain the oil well and add beeswax following the standard of about 1/4 cup grated beeswax per 1 cup of infused oil. Melt beeswax and pour into sterile containers. Rub this on your legs before you go to bed at night.

Valerian root will help for insomnia as well as restlessness. It will help with muscle restlessness.

Magnesium can relieve the spasms a person with restless leg syndrome might suffer from. It can also help with better sleep at night. Magnesium is responsible for over 300 bodily functions. It is so important for our body's. Magnesium deficiency has been directly linked to many things like ADHD, depression, anxiety, fibromyalgia, muscle spasms, insomnia, and on and on.

Women's Remedies

Women are complicated creatures, just ask any man! We go through so many different cycles in our lives, menstruation, fertility, child-bearing, and menopause. And with each of these different times, comes many complicated side effects due to hormonal fluctuations. We become super sensitive to internal and external things, and then we add in things like poor diet, no physical activity, and stress, and wow - we have a really complicated problem. We add in symptoms like food cravings, immune dysfunction, skin problems, breast tenderness, and more. Lucky for us, we have some great gifts from Mother Nature that can help us.

Menstrual Issues

Menstrual cramps and hot flashes **Female Balancing Formula** from "Herbal First Aid and Health Care"

Make a tincture from 100 proof Vodka or 60% vegetable glycerin and 40% water

2 parts each: Wild Yam Root, Angelica root, Chaste tree berries, Black Cohosh root

1 part each: Damiana leaf, hops flowers, licorice root, horsetail herb, motherwort herb

Take 1 - 2 dropperfuls as needed to help relieve symptoms

Menstrual Cramps

Black Cohosh, valerian, wild yam, yarrow, chamomile, and feverfew are herbs that have a reputation for easing menstrual cramps. Cramps can vary in large degree from person to person, so what works great for one woman will not necessarily work for another. Try these herbs and a few different combinations to really see what works best for your severity of cramps. I would recommend that you start drinking the tea or taking the capsules a day or two before you are expecting your cramps to start, and then during the first couple of days of the cramps, take every two hours as needed. Don't let it get ahead of you. Many ladies will wait until the cramps hit full force and then try to battle them. Be pro active and plan ahead.

Cramp bark is also useful to help ease cramps. It is a very potent antispasmodic and also affects the other organs besides the uterus. It works quickly to ease cramps. It has also been known to be used to halt early labor contractions, but always check with someone who knows more before taking powerful herbs during pregnancy.

Red Raspberry leaf tea is a great toner of the uterus and can also help prevent cramps. It needs to be taken over long periods of time to receive full benefits, and can be taken daily without any side effects as a general tonic during all pregnancy years.

Evening Primrose oil is an essential oil that is really strong and great for relieving PMS symptoms. Follow the instructions on the bottle of the oil and begin taking one week before your menstruation is to begin to gain full benefits.

Dong Quai is a great her for relieving menstrual complaints and menopausal symptoms. It is high in B12, and contains ferulic acid, which is a muscle relaxer and pain reliever. It shouldn't be taken by pregnant women, but then they don't fall into the category of menstruation or menopause.

Chaste Tree is a great herb to help with hormone regulation, as it act's directly on the pituitary gland. It increases your progesterone production which is directly linked to infertility, heavy bleeding, irregular periods, and PMS. It is a slow acting herb, but taken over several months it will show great results. Not for use by pregnant women.

Menopause

Let's face it, all of us ladies have to go through this at some point in our lives. It doesn't have to be a bad thing. Eating a healthy diet can go a long way to lessen the effects of menopause. Keeping our bodies healthy and functioning properly will ease symptoms and help us cope. Herbs can play a very important role long term in nourishing the body and female system, and there are a few things that we can do to get us through the symptoms that accompany menopause. For the purpose of this book, we are only going to consider a few of the symptoms and what some of the first aid remedies could be to help in a pinch.

Hot Flashes

Black Cohosh tincture can be beneficial to help relieve hot flashes in women. **Oregon grape root and dandelion root** also will help. These can be drank in a tea or used in capsule or tincture form.

Hot flash tea or capsule

1 part Black Cohosh

1 part Wild Sarsaparilla

1 part Hops

1 part Ginseng

This can be infused for a great tea, or if you would prefer capsule form, put all herbs in the blender and pulse until they are mixed and chopped fine together. Fill capsules. Take capsules as needed.

Mood Swings capsules

2 parts Vervain

1 part Wild Yam

1 part Chaste Tree Berry

1 part St. John's wort

1 part Peppermint or lemon balm

This formula can be blended together (using dry herbs) and then when it is blended fine, fill capsules. Take one or two capsules a couple of times a day as you feel you are having problems with mood swings. This will help to balance out the hormones and calm the nervous system.

Insomnia tea or capsules

2 parts Skullcap

1 part Passionflower

1 part Lemon Balm

1 part Nettle

Drinking a cup of tea or making these herbs into capsules and taking 2 or 3 before bed time, will help your nervous system relax enough that sleep should come easily. Hops could also be added into this formula add one part hops.

Ache Capsules

2 parts Gingko Biloba

2 parts Feverfew

1 part Black Cohosh

1 part Ashwaghanda

Make into capsules by blending all dry herbs in a blender together until they are fine. Make into capsules and take 2 capsules daily or a couple of times a day as needed to help alleviate head aches and body aches that come with menopause or perimenopause.

Whole Herb Tinctures

A tincture really can be a simple remedy. Most herbs have multiple properties and a simple tincture made with one herb can work wonders. Learning which herbs have which properties and being able to use one tincture for several different symptoms, that shows a great herbalist. It really doesn't have to be a complicated thing. It is really great if you have a selection of whole herb tinctures in your first aid kit, and you know what to do with them.

Whole Herb Tinctures

There are some good herbs to have on hand as individual tinctures. You can always combine them if you come across a recipe that calls for a blend.

Cayenne Pepper - good to help stop bleeding, fevers, varicose veins, asthma.

Dandelion root - brings quick relief to chronic inflammation of liver, relieves stomach cramps, helps to clear up skin rashes, among many other things. It is an all around nourishing tonic.

Nettle leaf - used for allergies, and anaemia. Great tonic and source of iron. Good for stimulating circulation.

Oregon Grape Root - great antiseptic and antibacterial, will lower fevers and fight infection, good liver tonic and detoxifier

Plantain herb - good for constipation or diarrhea. Use on bites and stings, including animal bites. Use on all external wounds. Good internal for asthma and bronchial

Skullcap herb - good tincture for nervous or anxiety, and insomnia. Best herb for with drawl symptoms from barbiturates and tranquilizers

St. John's wort - good for depression, anxiety, and nervous tension Good for shingles, bruises and injuries

Valerian - best for insomnia, anxiety, cramps, migraines, hypertension and painful menstruation

Wild yam root - used for irritable bowel syndrome, stomach complaints, morning sickness, painful menstruation, asthma and whooping cough

White Willow Bark - can replace aspirin for pain relief.

Yarrow flower and leaves - powerful healer and purifier, internally for fever and diarrhea and pretty much anything else. Yarrow is often considered a cure for all ills.

Essential Oils for First Aid

Essential Oils are a viable option for many conditions and should be considered as strong medicine. They should never be used straight on skin as they could cause irritation or an allergic reaction. Do you research and learn about them, using an open mind, and experiment to see what works best for your symptoms.

Lavender Oil: a great to use as a pain reliever or soothing and calming massage oil. When diluted and then rubbed into feet, temples, neck, or back to help one relax and get ready for sleep. It can be used as a decongestant through steam inhalation.

Eucalyptus Oil: An strong antiseptic, antiviral, and decongestant. It is good to use in steam inhalation to help relieve congestion in the throat, lungs, and sinus area. Good to do this for bronchitis and hay fever. It works great in a massage oil to be rubbed into the sinus, throat, or lung area, chest or back.

Tea Tree Oil: Diluted in a carrier oil is good to help treat athlete's foot. It is a really strong antiviral, antibacterial, and anti fungal. It can be used to treat congestion in the lungs or sinus by using it in a steam inhalation. It is strong enough to be used to treat Staphylococcus and many other fungal infections. Keep away from the area of the eyes because it can cause irritation.

Peppermint Oil: Great oil to use for indigestion and upset stomach. Dilute a little with a carrier oil and then rub into the abdomen to treat indigestion or IBS. Rubbed into the temples, painful joints and muscles it is effective to help relieve the aches.

Clove Oil: Is most often used as a natural pain killer for toothaches and infections. When combining with baking soda, and then rubbed onto the affected area of the tooth, it will cause temporary relief. It is a very strong oil so use sparingly

Arnica Oil: is used only topical for muscle injuries and aches. It is never to be taken internally or inhaled. Use only as a rub for painful muscles and joints.

Geranium Oil: has blood-clotting or hemostatic properties, and when applied to small wounds and cuts is can stop bleeding.

Helichrysum Oil: a strong analgesic and anti-inflammatory, used to treat arthritis, carpal tunnel syndrome, and fibromyalgia as a massage oil diluted in a carrier oil.

Rosemary Oil: antibacterial, anti-fungal, and anti-parasitic. Inhalation, cold or steamed, will help relieve congestion. Diluted in a carrier oil and used on temples, neck or tension areas can help relieve headaches and muscle aches.

Clary Sage Oil: Good for hormonal irregularities. Has a mild sedative effect when inhaled or massaged into feet or temples on head, or back.

Wintergreen Oil: a natural anticoagulant and analgesic. One oz of oil is equivalent to 171 aspirin if ingested, it is very strong.

Oregano Oil: a strong antiseptic, and antibacterial. Really great for topical applications for infections, but must be diluted with a carrier oil as it is really strong.

Thyme Oil: used to cure skin infections, and effective for ringworm and athlete's foot. Used as a steam inhalation for congestion in upper respiratory.

Disclaimer

The statements made in this book are my own opinions and ideas gathered through the years. They are not to be used in replace of diagnosis or treatments. They are not a cure for disease. They are to be used with caution and at your own discretion. I have made and used most of them and recommend them, however, am not responsible for any possible reactions that might come from them. Be wise as always. If in doubt on anything, please seek the advise of a physician or a naturopathic doctor, never guess or assume something, always look for answers.